EVIDENCE-BASED
ON CALL

ACUTE
MEDICINE
POCKETBOOK

*This book is dedicated to Kilgore Trout
and the Harrison sunflower.*

Commissioning Editor: Michael Parkinson
Project Development Manager: Jim Killgore
Project Manager: Nancy Arnott
Designer: Erik Bigland

EVIDENCE-BASED
ON CALL

ACUTE
MEDICINE
POCKETBOOK

Edited by

Christopher M. Ball MA (Cantab), BM BCh, MRCP
Project Director and Associate Research Fellow,
Centre for Evidence-based Medicine,
University of Oxford, Oxford, UK

Robert S. Phillips MA (Cantab), BM BCh, MRCPCH
Associate Research Fellow, Centre for Evidence-based Medicine,
University of Oxford and Specialist Registrar in Paediatrics,
Yorkshire Deanery, UK

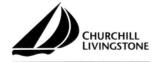

CHURCHILL
LIVINGSTONE

EDINBURGH LONDON NEW YORK PHILADELPHIA ST LOUIS SYDNEY
TORONTO 2002

CHURCHILL LIVINGSTONE
An imprint of Harcourt Publishers Limited

© Oxford Medical Knowledge 2002

 is a registered trademark of Harcourt Publishers Limited

First published 2002

ISBN 0443-07178-0

British Library Cataloguing in Publication Data
A catalogue record for this book is available from the
British Library

Library of Congress Cataloging in Publication Data
A catalog record for this book is available from the
Library of Congress

Note
Medical knowledge is constantly changing. As new
information becomes available, changes in treatment,
procedures, equipment and the use of drugs become
necessary. The editors and the publishers have taken
care to ensure that the information given in this text is
accurate and up to date. However, readers are
strongly advised to confirm that the information,
especially with regard to drug usage, complies with
the latest legislation and standards of practice.

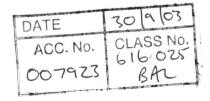
The
publisher's
policy is to use
**paper manufactured
from sustainable forests**

Printed in China

This book should really be called 'EBM at 2 a.m.'. It is a handbook about practical evidence-based medicine, offering support and an immediate answer when no other critically appraised resources are available.

In many ways it is similar to other handbooks – it is short and compact, and aimed at filling on-call pockets and mental voids. What makes it different is how it was written. We have gone back to the primary literature to try to validate every step of clinical management, and used evidence-based medicine techniques to select, appraise and summarize the material we have written. We have worked hard to separate fact from opinion, and rank everything we say for the quality of the material we've based it on. Where the evidence is weak, we have made recommendations based on our current clinical practice – these are not necessarily the best, just safe ones.

This book is deliberately (almost) number-free. There is a fatter version of this book[1] that contains a wealth of numbers and more detailed explanations; and there is also a website www.eboncall.co.uk that provides links to one-page summaries of the original articles on which we have based our recommendations. So you don't have to trust us – you can check it!

This book doesn't
- Give you all the answers.
- Tell you how to manage your patient. We have indicated the best management for most patients, but reckon only you (using your clinical expertise) and your patient (inputting their ideas and values) can decide what that best path might be.
- Guarantee drug doses or recipes – we have tried extremely hard to give accurate information for a typical adult patient, but encourage you to check your local formulary for more information.

It does give
- Some useful pointers and reminders, including drug recipes and some facts and figures that your patients might like to know.
- Some idea about the quality of the evidence for common clinical interventions. We have graded all our recommendations from A to D. Our grading reflects only the weight of evidence, not the clinical importance of the recommendation.[2]

---

1 Ball CM, Phillips RS *Evidence-based On-call Acute Medicine*, Churchill Livingstone 2001 (ISBN: 0-443-06412-1).

2 A cautionary note: these grades speak only to the validity of evidence about prevention, diagnosis, prognosis, therapy, and harm. Other strategies (see Sackett DL et al. *Evidence-based Medicine: how to practice and teach EBM*. Churchill Livingstone 2000 (ISBN: 0-443-06240-4)) must be applied to the evidence in order to generate clinically useful measures of its potential clinical implications and to incorporate vital patient-values into the ultimate decisions.

The ideas behind EBOC sprang from our personal struggles with understanding medicine and not knowing how to integrate the best evidence into our clinical practice. As a medical student, Chris Ball got labelled as 'boorish and vitriolic' for asking difficult questions. Fortunately Dave Sackett arrived from Canada, and showed him that evidence-based medicine offered a way of finding out the answers without getting lynched. On qualifying, Chris found some answers in a set of clinical guidelines that saved him and many a patient during his house officer year. However over time he became increasingly worried that they were getting out of date and weren't evidence-based. Together with Bob Phillips, he decided to pull these guides apart, find the evidence for every single recommendation, and then put them back together again. Having ripped apart general medicine, he is now deconstructing other specialties.

Bob Phillips practised 'evidence-based' medicine because he was sure there was no other way. After a year of carrying round a hundred critically appraised topics (CATs) on his Psion palmtop computer, and constantly being nagged by other clinicians for the information, Evidence-based On Call was a natural progression. With a care to focus on the patient, he is sure the application of the best available evidence has saved pain, distress and possibly lives.

We've worked hard at making each summary as accurate and practical as possible – nonetheless we're certain some errors, inaccuracies and confusion will have slipped in. If you spot any or can think of way to improve EBOC, e-mail us at eboncall@yahoo.com

If you want to find out more about more about practising and teaching EBM, we encourage you to grab the nearest copy of Evidence-based Medicine. Written by David Sackett and some of the other top EBM exponents, it provides a fun, rapid and easy introduction to some of these ideas. The book has an associated website at http://www.cebm.utoronto.ca, which provides more in-depth information. The Centre for Evidence-based Medicine's website at http://cebm.jr2.ox.ac.uk also provides teaching materials and information on courses.

CMB
RSP

ACKNOWLEDGEMENTS

This book springs from sharing diet Cokes and computer projectors with Dave Sackett and Muir Gray. Martin Dawes, Olive Goddard, and Douglas Badenoch at the Centre for Evidence-based Medicine at the University of Oxford have kept Bob and Chris academically respectable since then. Cheers guys.

We give special thanks to Lee Bailey, Musab Hayatli, Mary Hodgkinson and Clare Wotton who have worked in tiny rooms and under incredible pressure. Together with the gang at Oxford Medical Knowledge, their humour and patience have made EBOC lots of fun.

Without the funding of the BUPA Foundation and UK NHS Research and Development this project would not have happened. Equally Mike Parkinson and Jim Killgore at Harcourt-Brace have worked incredibly hard to create the final version – thanks to you all.

We thank our families for their love and our many colleagues who have offered advice and support as this project has developed. In particular we acknowledge Nick Shenker, Sharon Straus, Steve Hsu and Charles Pantin. This book is better because of you.

Euan A. Ashley BSc MBChB MRCP
Wellcome Trust Cardiovascular Research Fellow
Department of Cardiovascular Medicine
University of Oxford, John Radcliffe Hospital, Oxford, UK

Michael Bennett MB BS, FFARCSI, FANZCA, MM(Clin Epi)
Medical Director
Department of Diving and Hyperbaric Medicine
Prince of Wales Hospital, Randwick, Australia

Catherine M Clase BA, MB, BChir, MSc, FRCPC
Assisant Professor, Division of Nephrology
Dalhousie University, Halifax, Nova Scotia, Canada

Mary-Anne Cotton MB BS MRCPsych
University College Hospital, London, UK

Sumit Dhingra BA BM BCh
Oxford, UK

Robert Dinniwell MD
Ontario, Canada

John Epling MD
Assistant Professor of Family Medicine
Lafayette Family Medicine Residency and Center for Evidence-Based Practice
State University of New York - Upstate Medical University, Lafayette, NY, USA

David C. Ford MD MSc FRCP(C)
Division of Gastroenterology
McMaster University Canada

Carl Heneghan BA BM BCh
Oxford, UK

Richard Keatinge MRCGP
Wanfairpwll, UK

Warren L. Lee MD
Fellow in Respirology and Critical Care Medicine
University of Toronto, Canada

Geraldine Martell MBBS
Northampton, UK

Joel Ray MD
Toronto, Canada

Tim Ringrose MRCP
John Radcliffe Hospital, Oxford, UK

Nicholas Shenker MRCP
Specialist Registrar in Rheumatology
Whipps Cross Hospital, London, UK

Donald E. Stanley FCAP
Associate Professor of Pathology and Laboratory Medicine
Maine, USA

Matthew Taylor BA BM BCh
Department of General Medicine
John Radcliffe Hospital, Oxford, UK

Alain Townsend FRCP
IMM, John Radcliffe Hospital, Oxford, UK

Will Whiteley BM BCh
Whittington Hospital, London, UK

Ben Wong MD
Chief Medical Resident
Department of Internal Medicine
McMaster University, Canada

Ati Yates MD
Internal Medicine and Psychiatry
Anaconda Community Hospital, Montana, USA

EBM ADVISORY BOARD

Muir Gray FRCP
Director, National Electronic Library for Health
London, UK

David L Sackett MD
Director, Trout Research Centre and Conference Centre
Ontario, Canada

REVIEWERS

Anaemia
D. Chitnavas MRCP
Locum Consultant in Haematology
John Radcliffe Hospital
Oxford, UK

Anaphylaxis
Malcolm Daniel MRCP FRCA
Intensive Care Unit
Glasgow Royal Infirmary
Glasgow, Scotland

Unstable angina
I.K. Jang MD
Cardiology Division
Bulfinch 105, 55 Finch St
Boston, USA

Anticoagulation
A. Gallus MRCP & D. Keeling MRCP
John Radcliffe Hospital
Oxford, UK

Asthma exacerbation
B.R. O'Driscoll MRCP
Consultant Chest Physician
Hope Hospital
Salford, UK

Atrial fibrillation
R.G. Hart MD
Department of Medicine
University of Texas Health Science Center
San Antonio, Texas, USA

Bradyarrhythmias
B. McGovern MD
Boxford, MA, USA

Carbon monoxide poisoning
C.D. Scheinkestel FRCAP
Alfred Hospital
Melbourne, Victoria, Australia

Cellulitis
C. Conlon FRCP
John Radcliffe Hospital
Oxford, UK

Coma
Malcolm Daniel MRCP FRCA
Intensive Care Unit
Glasgow Royal Infirmary
Glasgow, Scotland

Congestive heart failure
B. Lee MD
Boston, USA

Exacerbation of COPD
N.R. Anthonisen MD
Faculty of Medicine
University of Manitoba
Winnipeg, Manitoba, Canada

Deep vein thrombosis
J. Ginsberg MD
McMaster University
Hamilton, Ontario, Canada

Diabetic ketoacidosis
N. Chi MD
Whitehead Institute
Nine Cambridge Center
Cambridge, MA, USA

Upper GI bleeding
L. Friedman MD
Massachusetts General Hospital,
Boston, MA, USA

Giant cell arteritis
M. V. Kyle FRCP
Department of General Medicine
Frenchay Hospital
Bristol, UK

Hypercalcaemia
S.B. Ramirez MD
Department of Paediatrics
National University Hospital
Singapore

Hyperkalaemia
C. Clase FRCPC
Division of Nephrology, Dalhousie
University
Halifax, Nova Scotia, Canada

Hypertensive crisis
S. Hsu MD
Department of Medicine
National University Hospital
Singapore

Hypoglycaemia
D. Matthews MRCP
Diabetes Centre
Radcliffe Infirmary
Oxford, UK

Hyponatraemia
J.V. Bonventre MD
Mass General Hospital-East
Department of Medicine
Charlestown, MA, USA

Infective endocarditis
E. Abrutyn MD
MCP Hahnemann School of Medicine
Philadelphia, PA, USA

Inflammatory bowel disease
L. Friedman MD
Massachusetts General Hospital
Boston, MA, USA

Meningitis
B. Davis MD
Massachusetts General Hospital
Boston, MA, USA

Pleural effusion
D. Geddes MRCP
Brompton Hospital
London, UK

Community-acquired pneumonia
M. Kamei MD
Nagoya-shi
Aichi, Japan

Pulmonary embolism
B. Lee MD
Boston, USA

Acute renal failure
S. Hsu MD
Dept. of Medicine
National University Hospital
Singapore

Sickle cell crisis
G. Serjeant MD
Medical Research Council Laboratories
Sickle Cell Unit
University of the West Indies
Kingston, Jamaica

Stroke
G. Donnan FRCAP
Head of Neurosciences
Austin & Repatriation Medical Centre
Heidelberg, Victoria, Australia

Syncope
W.N. Kapoor MD
Department of Medicine
University of Pittsburgh Medical Center
Pennsylvania, USA

Tachycardias
H. Oral MD
Department of Internal Medicine
University of Michigan Medical Center
Ann Arbor, USA

Other chapters reviewed by editorial team

CONTENTS

HOW TO USE THIS BOOK

This book is designed for clinicians who want or need to know the best available evidence in a hurry, so they can concentrate on using their own personal skills and expertise to care for their patients. It can be used by any clinician, at any stage of their training, to assist with decisions or prop up uneven table legs.

Evidence-based medicine is the conscientious, explicit and judicious use of current best evidence in making decisions about the care of individual patients. In keeping with this, each topic covered in *Evidence-based On Call* provides not a cookbook of what to do, but a series of recommendations about issues to consider when caring for your patients.

THE LAYOUT

Topics are arranged alphabetically, and indexed by disease area. Each topic is divided into sections based on clinical decisions; symptoms and signs, investigations, therapy, and ward review, with additional information on differential diagnosis and outcomes.

The grading (A, B, C, or D) after each recommendation reflects the weight of evidence in support of it (e.g. for therapeutic studies):

- A – randomized controlled trial (RCT) or review of RCTs, all-or-none data.
- B – cohort study, case-control study, poor RCT, or systematic review of cohort studies or case-control studies.
- C – care series, with no control group.
- D – expert opinion, physiology, bench research.

See Appendix I for a fuller explanation.

The layout does not reflect a set approach to caring for your patient – clearly if a patient is critically ill, therapeutic interventions may need to precede a detailed history and physical examination.

The bullet points in the 'symptoms and signs' and 'investigations' sections have been customized to provide more information about the related sign, symptom or test:

- A + symbol indicates that if the clinical feature is present or the investigation is abnormal, then the target disorder is more likely.
- A – symbol indicates that if the clinical feature is absent or the investigation is normal, then the target disorder is less likely.
- A ± symbol means the clinical feature or investigation can help diagnose and exclude the target disorder.
- A square (■) bullet point indicates that the clinical feature or investigation provides information about prognosis rather than diagnosis, or that there is not enough evidence to indicate whether it helps diagnose or exclude the target disorder.

THE PROBLEMS

There are two major deficits in this book. First – you have to trust the summary of the evidence we provide; there isn't physical space to give more supporting data! Second – it's out of date already as this was written in late 2000. To tackle the first problem, you can be reassured by the process we use to write the book, and assess the evidence we have found by looking at the critically appraised topics (CATs) – short summaries of the studies – available on the website at www.eboncall.co.uk. To address the second issue, we've put 'expiry dates' on all our material, and made up-to-date information available on the website (probably containing stuff that isn't published at the time we write!).

THE SOLUTIONS

The Evidence-Based On Call process takes important topics in clinical practice, turns them into a series of clinical questions, and answers them with the best evidence available. This is accomplished by two independent researchers performing searches first on the 'Best Evidence' CD-ROM, then in the Cochrane Library, Clinical Evidence, and finally the PubMed (www.ncbi.nlm.nih.gov/entrez/query.fcgi) database. The researchers' strategy is to look for high quality evidence in each database in order, only progressing to the next if no quality answer to their question is found. (The search terms they have used can be found appended to the foot of each CAT). The papers found are then appraised (using previously published criteria*) and summarized as critically appraised topics (or CATs). Each CAT is checked by an independent researcher for accuracy, and reviewed by an experienced clinician for validity and relevance, before being made available on the website. The CATs in turn are collated by a clinician and used to produce a topic guideline, which is in turn assessed by an experienced clinician before publication. Each article and each guide is then labelled with an expiry date.

The expiry dates reflect the inexorable advance of clinical medicine, and the realization that half of what we do now will be laughed at in 50 years' time (but we're never sure which half . . .). The material in this book is slowly decaying, and it will stink in 3 years' time (sooner in some cases). When the information hits its 'best before' date, the whole process of search, appraisal and review rolls over again to ensure the website contains the freshest evidence we can find.

In the between time though, the literature is constantly scanned by the review editor and the team of clinicians who support the Evidence-Based On Call process. If an important article is found, there is no waiting for an expiry date; the process of appraisal and review moves on and the updated information is introduced.

* Sackett DS et al.: *Clinical Epidemiology – a basic science for clinical medicine*; Little Brown (ISBN: 0-316-76599-6); the 'Users' guide to medical literature' section in JAMA running from 1992–97 available at http//:hiru.mcmaster.ca/ebm; and the policy and procedures from the journals *Evidence-based Medicine* and *ACP Journal Club*.

1
ALCOHOL WITHDRAWAL

SYMPTOMS AND SIGNS

Ask about:
- recent drink history including the number of drinks per day [C]
- ± the CAGE questions: [A]
  - have you ever attempted to **C**ut back on your drinking?
  - have you ever been **A**nnoyed at criticism about your drinking?
  - have you ever felt **G**uilty about drinking?
  - have you ever used alcohol as an **E**ye opener?
- other medical conditions [C]
- psychiatric symptoms [C]
- current medication, particularly frequent use of sedatives. [C]

> **CAGE questions**
> - Patients who answer 'yes' to three or more are very likely to have alcohol dependency.
> - Patients who answer 'no' to all four questions are unlikely to have alcohol dependency.

Look for:
- symptoms of withdrawal: [C]
  - nausea and vomiting
  - tremor
  - paroxysmal sweats
  - anxiety, agitation, confusion
  - tactile, visual or auditory disturbances
  - headache
- physical injury [D]
- Wernicke's encephalopathy [D] – ataxia, ophthalmoplegia and confusion
- Korsakoff's syndrome [D] – loss of recent memory, causing confabulation
- stigmata of chronic liver disease (see Chapter 13).

> **Think about**
> - Other causes of an acute confusional state.
> - Other drug withdrawal conditions.
> - Acute alcoholic hepatitis.

INVESTIGATIONS

- Blood count. [C]
- Clotting. [D]

- Ethanol level. [D]
- U&E, creatinine. [D]
- Glucose.[D]
+ Liver function tests [C] including gamma-GT. [C]

THERAPY

- Treat any dehydration, electrolyte imbalance or hypoglycaemia. [D]
- Give a benzodiazepine, preferably a long-acting one, [B] by mouth. [B]
- Consider offering patients a symptom-triggered regimen rather than a fixed schedule. [A]
- Give thiamine 100 mg daily for at least 2 days [C] by mouth or parenterally. [C]
- Give lorazepam 2 mg i.v. to patients who have had a seizure. [A]

A withdrawal regimen
- Fixed dose: give diazepam 10 mg three times a day, gradually reducing over the next few days, plus additional doses of 5 mg if your patient scores > 8 on the alcohol withdrawal scale (Table 1.1).
- Symptom-triggered: give diazepam 5 mg every time your patient scores > 8 on the alcohol withdrawal scale.
- Avoid long-acting benzodiazepines in patients with liver failure and give smaller doses less often. [D]

Note
- Patients with mild to moderate symptoms can be managed as outpatients [A] and patients with only mild withdrawal symptoms may not require any medication. [C]

REVIEW

- Monitor withdrawal symptoms using an alcohol withdrawal scale [A] – aim for a total score < 10 (Table 1.1).
- Advise patients to stop drinking. [A]
- Refer them to an alcoholism treatment clinic. [A] Send them a reminder letter to attend the clinic. [A]

Outcomes
- Delirium tremens and hallucinations are common. [A]
- Recurrent seizures are common [A] – anticonvulsants do not clearly help. [D]
- Many patients are drinking again within 2 weeks. [C]

Expires July 2003 Guideline: Richard Keatinge, Chris Ball
CATs: Richard Keatinge, Mary-Anne Cotton, Clare Wotton, Musab Hayatli, Chris Ball

Table 1.1 The Clinical Institute Withdrawal Assessment for Alcohol, Revised (CIWA-AR): sum the individual scores

Score	0	1	2
Temperature		37.0–37.5°C	37.5–38.0°C
Pulse (beats/min)		90–95	95–100
Respiration rate (per minute)		23–24	> 24
Blood pressure (diastolic mmHg)		95–100	100–103
Nausea and vomiting (do you feel sick, have you vomited?)	none		nausea with no vomiting
Tremor (arms extended, fingers spread)	no tremor		not visible – can be felt fingertip to fingertip
Sweating (observation)	no sweat visible		barely perceptible, palms moist
Tactile disturbances	none		mild itching, or pins and needles or numbness
Auditory hallucinations (loud noises, hearing voices)	not present		mild harshness or ability to frighten (increased sensitivity)
Visual disturbances (photophobia, seeing things)	not present		mild sensitivity (bothered by lights)
Hallucinations	none	auditory, tactile or visual only	non-fused auditory or visual
Clouding of sensorium (what day is this? what place is this?)	orientated		disorientated for date by no more than 2 days
Quality of contact	in contact with examiner		seems in contact, but oblivious to environment
Anxiety (do you feel nervous?) (observation)	no anxiety; at ease		appears anxious
Agitation (observation)	normal activity		somewhat more than normal activity
Thought disturbances (flight of ideas)	no disturbance		does not have much control over nature of thoughts
Convulsions, (seizures or fits of any kind)	no		
Headache (does it feel like a band around your head?)	not present		mild
Flushing of face	none	mild	severe

3	4	5	6
> 38.0°C			
100–105	105–110	110–120	> 120
103–106	106–109	109–112	> 112
	intermittent nausea with dry heaves		nausea, dry heaves, vomiting
	moderate with arms extended		severe even with arms not extended
	beads of sweat visible		drenching sweats
	intermittent tactile hallucinations (e.g. bugs crawling)		continuous tactile hallucinations
	intermittent auditory hallucinations (appears to hear things you cannot)		continuous auditory hallucinations (shouting, talking to unseen persons)
	intermittent visual hallucinations (occasionally seeing things you cannot)		continuous visual hallucinations (seeing things constantly)
fused auditory and visual			
disorientated for date	disorientated for place (reorientate if necessary)		
	periodically becomes detached		makes no contact with examiner
	moderately anxious or guarded		overt anxiety (equal to panic)
	moderately fidgety and restless		pacing, or thrashing about constantly
	plagued by unpleasant thoughts constantly		throughts come quickly and in a disconnected fashion
			yes
	moderately severe		severe

2
ANAEMIA

SYMPTOMS AND SIGNS

Ask about:
- recent bleeds [A,B]
- recent onset pallor [C]
- menstrual loss [B]

- diet and alcohol use [B,C]
+ weight loss (> 7 kg in 6 months) [C]

- family history of anaemia [D]
+ history of gastrectomy (if suspected vitamin B_{12} deficiency) [B] or other bowel resection [C]
+ upper gastrointestinal symptoms [C] (dysphagia, heartburn, nausea, vomiting)
+ lower gastrointestinal symptoms [C] (altered bowel habit, rectal bleeding, pain relieved by defecation).

Common causes of anaemia in the elderly [A,B]
- anaemia of chronic disease
- iron-deficiency anaemia
- recent bleeding
- vitamin B_{12} or folate deficiency
- myelodysplastic syndrome and acute leukaemia
- chronic leukaemia, lymphoma-related disorders
- other haematological disorders (myelofibrosis, aplastic anaemia, haemolytic anaemia)
- multiple myeloma.

Look for:
+ conjunctival pallor [A]
+ facial pallor [B]
+ palmar pallor [B]

Conjunctival pallor
Little or no evidence of red colour on anterior rim matching the fleshy part of the posterior aspect of the palpebral conjunctiva.

- evidence of acute bleeding [B]
+ supine tachycardia (pulse > 100 beats/min)
+ supine hypotension (systolic blood pressure < 95 mmHg)
+ postural pulse increase of ≥ 30 beats/min or severe dizziness on sitting upright, or on standing

Note
- Postural hypotension (a fall in systolic blood pressure > 20 mmHg on standing) does not usefully diagnose acute blood loss. [B]
- Patients can lose up to 600 ml of blood acutely without a supine tachycardia. [B]

■ evidence of heart failure [D]
■ jaundice (suggesting haemolytic or megaloblastic anaemia) [D]
■ evidence of infection or spontaneous bruising (suggesting marrow failure) [D]
■ abdominal or rectal masses [D]

+ Perform a rectal examination [D] and a faecal occult blood test. [A]

Note
The following are little help in diagnosing anaemia: [C]
- fatigue
- dizziness or palpitations
- angina
- a painful tongue
- diarrhoea or recent constipation.

INVESTIGATIONS

■ Blood count [A] and blood film. [A]
■ Group and save. [D]
■ Urea and electrolytes. [D]
■ Liver function tests. [D]

Mean cell volume and red cell distribution width results
Combining the MCV and RDW results can help define potential causes of the anaemia. [B]

MCV	RDW	Potential causes [B]
Low	Normal	Chronic disease, heterogenous thalassaemia
Low	High	Iron deficiency, RBC fragmentation (artificial valve), HbH, S beta-thalassaemia
Normal	Normal	Any chronic disease (including chronic liver disease), haemorrhage, haemolysis, transfusion, HbAS, HbAC, CLL with < 150 × 10^3 WBC/L, hereditary spherocytosis
Normal	High	Early iron or folate (or both) deficiency, HbSS, HbSC, myelofibrosis, sideroblastic anaemia
High	Normal	Aplastic anaemia, preleukaemia
High	High	Folate or B_{12} deficiency, immune haemolytic anaemia, cold agglutinins with > 150 × 10^9 WBC/L

Take the following tests before giving a blood transfusion. [A]

Microcytic anaemia
± Serum ferritin. [A]

Macrocytic anaemia
- Serum folate. [D]
- Serum B_{12} (cobalamin). [B]
± Urine methylmalonic acid (MMA) [B] or serum MMA [B] (if B_{12} deficiency suspected).

Further investigations
Iron-deficiency anaemia
- Gastroscopy and colonoscopy. [C]

Vitamin B_{12} deficiency
+ Intrinsic factor antibodies. [C]
+ Schilling test. [C]

Iron-deficiency anaemia
Two-thirds of cases are due to upper gastrointestinal disease. [B]
Common causes in the elderly include: [B]
- peptic ulcer disease or erosions
- colorectal neoplasia
- gastric surgery
- hiatus hernia (> 10 cm)
- upper GI malignancy
- angiodysplasia
- oesophageal varices.

Vitamin B_{12} deficiency
Common causes include: [C]
- pernicious anaemia
- tropical sprue
- bowel resection
- jejunal diverticula
- B_{12} malabsorption
- vegetarianism.

Folate deficiency

Common causes include: [C]
- alcoholism
- malnutrition.

THERAPY

Folate deficiency

■ Dietary assessment. [D]
- Treat acute GI bleeding (see Chapter 41).
- Treat congestive heart failure (see Chapter 21).
- In general, chronic anaemias do not require transfusion, unless the patient is symptomatic (when blood should be given slowly). [D]

Iron-deficiency anaemia

- Give iron supplements, [B] e.g. oral ferrous sulphate 200 mg three times a day. [D] Watch for constipation. [B]

Macrocytic anaemia

- Give hydroxycobalamin [A] 1 mg i.m. alternate days for 6 days. [D]
- Give folate 5 mg orally twice a day. [A]

Continue both until the results of vitamin assays are available, then treat as required. [A]

Other haematological disorders

- Discuss with a haematologist. [D]

Expires July 2004   Guideline: Chris Ball, Rob Dinniwell
CATs: Rob Dinniwell, Chris Ball

3
ANAPHYLAXIS

SYMPTOMS AND SIGNS

Symptoms of anaphylaxis vary, but commonly include: [C]
- swelling or angioedema
- wheeze, dyspnoea
- hypotension, arrhythmias
- pruritus
- diarrhoea, vomiting.

> **Causes of anaphylaxis** [C]
> - food, especially nuts
> - bites or stings
> - drugs or vaccines, especially
>   - antibiotics
>   - NSAIDs
>   - muscle relaxants
>   - contrast media.

Ask about:
- previous episodes of anaphylaxis [C]
- known allergies [A]
- a history of asthma or atopy [C]
- current medication. [A]

> **Think about other causes of collapse**
> - syncope
> - myocardial infarction
> - pulmonary embolism
> - hypovolaemia
> - overdose
> - aspiration.

THERAPY

- Assess airway, breathing and circulation rapidly.
- Give adrenaline 1:1000 1 ml i.m. (1 mg). [A]
- Scrape or pinch off wasp or bee stings [D] – don't leave them in!

Consider giving:
- i.v. fluid [A]
- salbutamol 5 mg [D] nebulizers if wheezy

- steroids [D]
- antihistamines. [D]

Monitor cardiac and respiratory function. [C]

REVIEW

- Educate your patient about the signs and symptoms of a recurrent attack, and known common triggers. [D]
- For patients with recurrent or severe attacks, arrange for:
  - skin prick or IgE testing [C]
  - a medical alert bracelet/card/letter [A]
  - an autoinjector of adrenaline for the patient to carry at all times. [A]

Consider prophylactic steroids for severe idiopathic cases. [C]

> **Outcome**
> - Death is uncommon for patients who are treated appropriately. [C]
> - One in 15 patients has a biphasic response with symptoms recurring 12 to 24 hours later [C] – warn patients about this.
> - Recurrent episodes often occur. [C]

4
AORTIC DISSECTION

SYMPTOMS AND SIGNS

Consider aortic dissection in all patients with chest or upper abdominal pain [C] especially if they:
- − have a history of hypertension [C]
- + have Marfan syndrome [C]
- + are pregnant. [D]

> **Think about other causes of chest pain** [C]
> - myocardial infarction
> - aortic regurgitation
> - thoracic non-dissecting aneurysm
> - musculoskeletal pain
> - mediastinal cyst or tumour
> - pericarditis
> - gallstones
> - pleuritis
> - pulmonary embolism.

Ask about:
- + chest pain [C] and if it has moved [C]
- − symptoms for < 24 hours. [C]

Look for:
- ± hypertension or hypotension [C]
- + absent or reduced pulses [C]
- + aortic regurgitation [C]
- ■ evidence of: [B]
  - ■ a myocardial infarction
  - ■ a stroke or paralysis
  - ■ renal failure.

> **Note**
> - No individual sign or symptom is very helpful in diagnosing aortic dissection.

INVESTIGATIONS

- ■ Blood count. [D]
- ■ Group and save. [D]
- ■ Cardiac enzymes. [B]
- ■ Urea and electrolytes, creatinine. [B]

- ECG. [C]
+ Chest X-ray. [B]

> **ECG changes**
> Look for:
> - myocardial infarction [D]
> + left ventricular hypertrophy. [C]

> **Chest X-ray changes**
> Look for: [B]
> - widening of the aorta (particularly the aortic knob) or mediastinum
> - a pleural effusion
> - tracheal shift.

Perform further imaging if an aortic dissection is still possible [D] in consultation with a cardiothoracic surgeon: [D]
± MRI [A]
± transoesophageal echocardiography (TOE). [A]

If these are not available:
+ CT thorax [A]
+ transthoracic echocardiography (TTE). [A]

> **Note**
> CT and transthoracic echocardiography cannot safely exclude an aortic dissection.

THERAPY

- Give analgesia [D] e.g. diamorphine 5 mg i.v. (in small or elderly patients 2.5 mg).
- Discuss with a cardiothoracic surgeon (and cardiologist) and organize transfer to a cardiothoracic unit or intensive care unit. [D]

> **Treatment options**
> Consider surgery [A] for patients with: [D]
> - acute dissection of the ascending aorta
> - acute dissection of the descending aorta with:
>   - signs of impending rupture (persisting pain, hypotension, left-sided haemothorax)
>   - Marfan syndrome
> - chronic dissection, if aorta > 5–6 cm in diameter or symptoms.
>
> Consider medical therapy (long-term antihypertensive therapy) for patients with acute or chronic dissection of the descending aorta. [D]

Meanwhile give antihypertensive therapy. [D] Options include:

- labetolol i.v.
- nitroprusside and propranolol i.v.
- trimetaphan i.v.

Labetalol

- Make up 200 mg labetalol in 200 ml 0.9% saline.
- Start an infusion at 0.25 mg/min (15 ml/h), increasing it every 15 min to a maximum total dose of 200 mg.

Nitroprusside

- Make up 50 mg nitroprusside in 500 ml 5% glucose.
- Start an infusion at 10 μg/min (6 ml/h), increasing it every 5 min in steps of 10 μg/min to a maximum of 75 μg/min (45 ml/h).

Consider inserting:

- an intra-arterial line for constant BP monitoring if using nitroprusside or trimetaphan [D]
- a urinary catheter. [D]

Aim for systolic blood pressure of 100–120 mmHg provided the urine output > 30 ml/hour. [D]

Outcomes

- Around a sixth die before surgery, many from aortic rupture. [B]
- Most survive surgery, though half are dead within 10 years. [B]
- One in 10 require further surgery within 7 years [B] – often for aortic rupture. [C]

5
ASTHMA EXACERBATION

SYMPTOMS AND SIGNS

Ask about:
- a previous history of asthma [B]
- severity of asthma:
    - normal peak expiratory flow rate [D] and whether it feels worse than normal [C]
    - any life-threatening asthma attacks (respiratory arrests or intubations) [B]
    - number of emergency department visits in the last 6 months [A]
    - any hospital admission within 12 months [B] or recent discharge from hospital [A]
- recent symptoms such as wheezing, [B] cough, [B] and dyspnoea, particularly on exertion
- current medication and its use [B]
- triggers for attacks [D]
- any psychosocial problems. [B]

> **Other causes of dypsnoea**
> - congestive heart failure
> - COPD
> - arrhythmia
> - infection
> - interstitial lung disease
> - anaemia
> - pulmonary embolism.

Look for:
- evidence of airway obstruction: [B]
    + wheezing
    + barrel chest
    + hyperresonance
    + forced expiratory time (> 9 seconds)
- signs of severity: [B]
    + moderate–severe dyspnoea
    + pulse ≥ 120 beats per minute
    + respiratory rate ≥ 30 per minute
- evidence of hypercapnia: [C]
    + a quiet chest
    + too dyspnoeic to talk
    + cyanosis
    + requiring supplemental oxygen
    − beta-agonists use

- accessory muscle use
- psychiatric symptoms or denial. C

> **Note**
> Pulsus paradoxus is not very helpful at diagnosing or ruling out severe asthma. B

INVESTIGATIONS

- Peak expiratory flow rate (PEFR). C
- Pulse oximetry. C
- Arterial blood gases, C using local anaesthetic. A

> **Note**
> - Neither clinicians nor patients accurately judge peak flows. C
> - Peak flows alone cannot safely exclude hypercapnia or hypoxia. C

After therapy, repeat:
- PEFR C
- arterial blood gases. C

Consider a chest X-ray if the following are present: C
- history of fever or temperature > 37.8°C
- heart disease
- i.v. drug misuse
- seizures
- immunosuppression
- other pulmonary disease
- previous thoracic surgery.

THERAPY

- Give oxygen 40–60%. D
- Give a beta-agonist A (e.g. salbutamol 2.5 to 5 mg) with an anticholinergic A (e.g. ipratropium 500 μg) via a nebulizer or an inhaler and holding chamber regularly A (and continuously if possible A) using air or oxygen. D
- Give steroids A immediately A in doses equivalent to 40 mg prednisolone daily A by any route. D

If patients are not improving, consider adding any of:
- aminophylline i.v. A
- salbutamol i.v. A (5 μg/min initially, adjusted to response up to 20 μg/min)
- magnesium sulphate 1.0 to 1.2 g intravenously over 30 minutes A
- adrenaline subcutaneously A 0.3 ml of 1:1000
- anaesthetic drugs. A

Aminophylline
- Arrange ECG monitoring.
- Add 250 ml to 500 ml of 0.9% saline.
- Give a loading dose of 5.6 mg/kg (2.8 ml/kg) over 20 min (not if patient has received aminophylline or oral theophylline in last 24 hours), followed by continuous infusion 0.9 mg/kg (0.45 ml/kg) per hour.
- Monitor theophylline levels [A] daily (therapeutic range 10–20 mg/L).
- Watch for features of toxicity (e.g. nausea, vomiting, arrhythmias).

Salbutamol
- Arrange ECG monitoring.
- Add 5 mg salbutamol to 500 ml 0.9% saline.
- Infuse at 3 to 20 µg/min (18 ml/h to 120 ml/h); start at 5 µg/min (30 ml/h).
- Watch for features of toxicity (e.g arrhythmias, hypokalaemia).

Consider admitting patients with a PEFR:
- < 100 L/min before therapy or < 300 L/min after therapy [C]
- < 50% predicted. [D]

Refer for **intubation and ventilation** if any of the following are present: [D]
- worsening peak flows
- worsening hypoxia or hypercapnia
- exhaustion or confusion
- coma or respiratory arrest.

REVIEW

- Continue oral [A] and inhaled [A] steroids for 3 to 10 days (e.g. 40 mg prednisolone daily, and inhaled budesonide 800 µg twice daily). Oral steroids can be stopped abruptly without tapering. [D]
- Check your patient's inhaler technique. [D]
- Provide an action plan and a peak flow meter. [A]
- Provide information on asthma for high-risk patients. [A]

Patients who improve can be discharged if:
- PEFR > 300 L/min and > 60% predicted and improving [C]
- any diurnal variation ≤ 20% predicted PEFR [D]
- they are symptom-free. [D]

Action plan [A]
If the PEFR is:
- ≤ 70% or ≥ 20% diurnal variation – double inhaled steroid dose
- ≤ 50% – steroid course
- ≤ 30% – seek urgent treatment.

Outcomes
- Relapses are common – half have another exacerbation within 8 weeks. [A]
- Few patients die, [B] even patients who require ventilation. [C]

Expires July 2003   Guideline: Chris Ball, Benny Wong
CATs: Chris Ball, Clare Wotton, Benny Wong

6
UNSTABLE ANGINA AND NON-Q WAVE MYOCARDIAL INFARCTION

SYMPTOMS AND SIGNS

Ask about:
- the pain, specifically:
  - its position, [B] looking for:
    + retrosternal chest pain [B]
  - its duration, [A] looking for:
    + chest pain which started ≥ 48 hours ago [A]
    + constant pain [B]
  - its nature, [A] looking for:
    + pressure [A]
    − no sharp or stabbing pain [A]
    − no pleuritic pain [A]
    − no positional pain [A]
  + any similarity to previous infarcts or angina attacks [A]
  - any exacerbating or relieving factors, [B] particularly:
    + pain brought on by exertion
    + pain relieved by nitrates or rest

+ a history of angina or MI [A]

- cardiovascular risk factors:
  - hypertension [A]
  - smoking [B]
  - diabetes mellitus [A]
  - elevated total cholesterol or triglycerides. [A]

Look for:
− absence of chest pain that is reproduced on palpation. [A]

Unstable angina

Defined as:
- angina for < 1 month with increasing severity, frequency or duration
- a sudden worsening of previously stable angina without change in medical therapy
- prolonged pain > 10 minutes or recurrent angina at rest.

With evidence of ischaemic heart disease – any of:
- previous myocardial infarction or angina
- transient ECG changes (ST depression or T wave inversion > 2 leads, ST depression, hyperacute T waves or both)
- positive exercise test or angiography.

Other common causes of chest pain include: C
- myocardial infarction
- pulmonary embolism
- chest infection
- musculoskeletal pain
- pericarditis.

Rarer causes include: D
- aortic dissection
- oesophageal spasm
- oesophageal rupture
- abdominal pain
  - gallstones
  - gastritis
- herpes zoster.

Estimate your patient's risk of significant coronary artery disease (> 50% coronary artery stenosis in at least one major artery – Tables 6.1, 6.2) using age [A] and the following symptoms: [B]

+ retrosternal chest pain
+ pain brought on by exertion
+ pain relieved in < 10 minutes by rest or GTN.

Table 6.1   MEN: probability of ≥ 50% coronary artery stenosis in at least one major artery

Age	30–39	40–49	50–59	60–69
Asymptomatic (0 symptoms)	2%	6%	10%	12%
Non-anginal chest pain (1 symptom)	5%	14%	22%	28%
Atypical angina (2 symptoms)	22%	46%	59%	67%
Typical angina (all 3 symptoms)	70%	87%	92%	94%

Table 6.2   Women: probability of ≥ 50% coronary artery stenosis in at least one major artery

Age	30–39	40–49	50–59	60–69
Asymptomatic (0 symptoms)	0.3%	1%	3%	8%
Non-anginal chest pain (1 symptom)	1%	3%	8%	19%

Table 6.2 *(Continued)*

Age	30–39	40–49	50–59	60–69
Atypical angina (2 symptoms)	4%	14%	32%	54%
Typical angina (all 3 symptoms)	26%	55%	79%	91%

INVESTIGATIONS

- Blood count. [D]
- U&E, creatinine. [D]
- Glucose. [A]
- Serial cardiac enzymes:
  - ± CK-MB over 24 hours [C]
  - ± troponin T [C]
  - ± creatinine kinase [B] over 48 hours with:
    - + lactate dehydrogenase. [A]
- Lipid levels. [A]
- ± 12-lead ECG, [A] followed by serial ECGs. [B]
- Chest X-ray. [D]

Cardiac enzymes
- An early CK-MB rise diagnoses a myocardial infarction and normal levels at 20 hours rule it out. [C]
- A normal troponin T or troponin I at 20 hours makes an infarct unlikely. [G]
- Elevated creatinine kinase levels [B] or an elevated myoglobin [C] diagnoses an infarct.
- CK, AST or LDH taken on presentation cannot safely diagnose or exclude an infarct. [A]

ECG
- Look for features suggesting cardiac ischaemia:
  - any ST elevation in 2 or more leads [A]
  - any ST depression [B]
  - any Q waves [A]
  - any T wave inversion [B]
  - any conduction defect. [B]
- These are more significant if present in 2 or more leads, or not known to be old.
- A normal ECG makes life-threatening complications unlikely. [C]

THERAPY

- Consider admitting your patient to a chest pain observation unit. [D]

Patients at low risk for a myocardial infarction

Patients can be assessed in a rapid evaluation unit by: [D]
- CK-MB at 0, 4, 8, 12 hours
- serial 12-lead ECGs
- clinical assessment at 0, 6, 12 hours
- exercise ECG: if all the above are negative.

- Treat symptoms rather than ECG changes. [D]
- Give oxygen. [D]
- Give aspirin [A] 300 mg orally, [D] then 75 mg daily; [A] alternatives include clopidogrel [A] 525 mg daily, then 75 mg daily;
  - with a low-molecular weight heparin (LMWH) [A] for as long as possible, e.g. enoxaparin s.c. 1 mg/kg twice daily. [A]
- For severe cases with ECG changes or cardiac enzyme elevation, give heparin with a glycoprotein IIb/IIIa inhibitor, e.g. eptifibatide [A] or tirofiban. [A]
- Consider starting anticoagulation (adjusted so INR is 2.2. to 2.5). [A]
- Give i.v. or buccal glyceryl trinitrate for chest pain. Consider adding long-acting nitrates. [C]
- Start:
  - a beta-blocker, [A] e.g. metoprolol 25 mg three times a day, or atenolol 50 mg daily, or
  - a calcium-channel blocker, e.g. diltiazem [A] 180 mg daily, or verapamil [A] 80 to 120 mg three times a day.
- For patients already on a beta-blocker, add a calcium channel blocker, [A] and vice versa. [A]

Heparin

- Add 25 000 units heparin to 50 ml 0.9% saline.
- Give a bolus, followed by an infusion using a weight-based nomogram.
- Check aPTT 6 hours later. Aim for an aPTT ratio of 1.5 to 2.5.

See Chapter 19 for more details on heparin dosing.

Glyceryl trinitrate

- 50 mg glyceryl trinitrate in 50 ml 0.9% saline.
- Give 1 to 10 mg/ml (1 to 10 ml) per hour.
- Titre to:
  - chest pain
  - systolic BP > 90 mmHg
  - headache.

For patients with severe refractory unstable angina, consider:
- adding a glycoprotein IIb/IIIa inhibitor [A]
- adding nicorandil [A] 10 mg twice daily
- angiography and revascularization. [A]

Alternatives include:
- thoracic epidural anaesthesia [A]
- adding n-acetylcysteine to nitrates. [A]

Need for coronary care unit admission

Use the following clinical prediction rule (Table 6.3) to help you determine whether your patient needs admission to a coronary care unit. [A]

Look for the following risk factors: [A]
- pain worse than prior angina or similar to pain associated with a previous infarction
- systolic blood pressure < 110 mmHg
- crackles above the bases bilaterally
- ST elevation or Q waves, not known to be old, in 2 or more leads
- ST segment or T wave changes, not known to be old, indicating myocardial ischaemia.

Table 6.3   Risk of major complications

Group	Risk of major complication within 4 days
Suspected MI, or ischaemia on ECG, or suspected and ≥ 2 risk factors	16%
Suspected ischaemia on ECG and ≥ 1 risk factor	8%
1 risk factor with no MI, or ischaemia on ECG	4%
No risk factors	0.5%

REVIEW

- Repeat cardiac enzymes [A] and ECGs [A] daily for at least 2 days. [D]
- Monitor for thrombocytopenia. [A]

Ask about:
- further chest pain [A]
- dyspnoea [A]
- palpitations. [A]

Look for: [B]
- arrhythmias
- new murmurs or a pericardial rub [B]
- signs of heart failure. [B]

Start:

- an ACE inhibitor [A] for patients with one other cardiovascular risk factor (hypertension, hypercholesterolaemia, low HDL levels, smoking or documented microalbuminuria). [A]

ACE inhibitors
- Monitor the blood pressure for the first dose. [D]
- Increase the dose if patients tolerate it. [A]
- Typical doses:
  - Enalapril 2.5 to 5 mg daily initially, increasing to 10 to 20 mg daily.
  - Perindopril 1 mg daily initially, increasing to 4 to 8 mg daily.
  - Ramipril 1.25 mg daily initially, increasing to 5 mg daily. [A]
- Monitor the renal function. [A]

Target cardiac risk factors:

- Encourage patients to stop smoking [A] and ask nurses [A] and other staff [A] to provide further advice. Offer:
  - nicotine patches [A] or gum [A]
  - buproprion. [A]
- Treat hypertension. [A]
- Optimize diabetes control. [A]
- Lower cholesterol levels [A] even for patients with average levels (cholesterol 4.0 to 6.2 mmol/L) [A] using:
  - diet modification; [A] encourage patients to eat a Mediterranean-style diet [A]
  - a statin [A]
  - gemfibrozil 600 mg twice daily for patients with low HDL levels. [A]
- Consider giving patients vitamin E supplements [A] 400 mg daily.

Dietary advice
- Eat more bread, more root and green vegetables, fish, and oats. [A]
- Eat less meat – replace beef, lamb, pork with poultry.
- Have no day without fruit.
- Replace butter and cream with margarine, rapeseed and olive oils.
- Eat more soy protein. [B]

Statins
- Start at a low dose and increase to the maximum tolerated: [D]
  - atorvastatin 40 mg at night
  - pravastatin 40 mg at night
  - simvastatin 40 mg at night.

Outcomes
- One in 30 has an MI within 3 weeks, [A] and one in 20 is dead within 6 weeks though the risk is higher with new-onset angina at rest or prolonged chest pain. [B]
- A fifth to a third require coronary revascularization within 3 years. [A]

Stress-testing

Perform stress-testing before discharge or as an outpatient [D] using any of:

- ± a symptom-limited [C] exercise tolerance test [A]
- ± myocardial perfusion scanning [A] looking for a reversible perfusion defect [B]
- ± exercise SPECT (single photon emission CT) [A]
- ± exercise echocardiography. [A]

Exercise ECG

Look for: [B]

- horizontal or down-sloping ST slope and 1 mm or more of depression in any lead
- angina during the test
- limited exercise duration
- impaired systolic blood pressure changes
- signs of poor ventricular function: ejection fraction < 40%.

Use the following clinical prediction rule to rank your patient for risk of dying. [A]

Total score = $D - (5 \times M) - (4 \times T)$

where: D = duration of exercise in minutes
M = maximal ST-segment deviation during or after exercise in mm
T = treadmill angina index (Table 6.4).

Table 6.4   Treadmill angina index

Angina during stress-testing	Score
Test stopped because of angina	2
Non-limiting angina	1
No angina	0

Interpretation of the total score is shown in Table 6.5.

Table 6.5   Assessing stress-test total score

Total score	Risk of dying within 4 years
< −10	High (20%)
−10 to +5	Moderate (5%)
≥ +5	Low (1%)

Refer all patients for coronary angiography (followed by PTCA or CABG as required) if they develop:

- spontaneous angina occurring > 36 hours after admission [A]

- prolonged angina with an ischaemic ECG
- abnormal stress testing [A]
- moderate to severe angina after hospital discharge despite maximal anti-ischaemic therapy. [A]

Angioplasty

Offer angioplasty to patients with single vessel disease. [B]

- Give a glycoprotein antagonist, e.g. abciximab, and insert a stent. [A]
- Following stent insertion give clopidogrel 75 mg once daily for one month. [A]
- Consider giving probucol. [A]

Angiography and angioplasty

Warn patients about the possibility of:

- death (3%)
- myocardial infarction (~5%)
- emergency bypass (2%)
- bleeding
- pseudoaneurysm formation
- renal failure from contrast dye (see Ch 19 for prophylaxis).

Coronary artery bypass surgery

Offer coronary artery bypass surgery to patients with:

- 3 vessel disease or left main artery disease [A]
- poor left ventricular function [A]
- severe angina [A]
- an abnormal exercise tolerance test. [A]

Coronary artery bypass surgery

- One in 30 dies within 1 month of bypass surgery.
- Patients take roughly 5 weeks longer to return to work than those having angioplasty. [A]

Offer spinal cord stimulation surgery to patients with severe angina, who are unsuitable for angioplasty but at high risk for coronary artery bypass grafting. [A]

7
ATRIAL FIBRILLATION

SYMPTOMS AND SIGNS

Look for:
+ an irregular pulse. [B]

Measure the rate using the apical pulse. [D]

Look for evidence of:
- heart disease:
    - ischaemic heart disease
    - congestive heart failure
    - valvular heart disease
    - cardiomyopathy
    - hypertension
- lung disease:
    - COPD
    - pulmonary embolism
- thyrotoxicosis [A]
- cardiovascular compromise: [D]
    - hypotension
    - heart failure.

Causes of atrial fibrillation include:
- ischaemic heart disease [A]
- cardiomyopathy [A]
- congestive heart failure [A]
- valvular heart disease [A]
- hyperthyroidism [A]
- alcohol [B]
- pulmonary disease [B] including PE.

INVESTIGATIONS

- Blood count. [D]
- U&E, creatinine. [D]
- Calcium, magnesium. [D]
- Cardiac enzymes. [D]
- Thyroid function tests. [A]
- 12-lead ECG. [A]
- Chest X-ray. [D]

Consider performing an echocardiogram. [A]

> **Echocardiogram**
> Look for:
> - global left ventricular dysfunction [A]
> - an enlarged left atrium [A]
> - occult mitral stenosis. [D]

THERAPY

Acute onset atrial fibrillation

Control the ventricular rate [A] using:
- Digoxin. [A]

> **Digoxin**
> - Load patients with 500 to 1000 μg in divided doses.
> - Give 62.5 to 250 μg daily, based on age, renal function and other medication.
> - Measure digoxin levels after 5 days. [D] Take the blood test 6 to 10 hours after the last dose.
> - Therapeutic range 0.8 to 2.0 ng/ml.

Alternatives include:
- Calcium-channel blockers:
  - verapamil 5 mg i.v. over 5 minutes; repeat after 5 minutes to a maximum dose of 20 mg
  - diltiazem 0.25 mg/kg over 2 minutes; repeat at 0.35 mg/kg if no response. [A]

- Beta-blockers:
  - esmolol: [A]
    - load patients with 100 μg/kg/min i.v. over 1 minute
    - followed by 50 μg/kg/min over 4 minutes
    - repeat if there is no effect, and increase the 4 minute infusion by 50 μg/kg/min
  - sotalol: [A]
    - 100 mg i.v. over 5 minutes, or 80 mg orally twice daily.

- Clonidine [B] 100 μg orally twice daily.

Consider cardioversion [A] if your patient fails to revert spontaneously. [D]

Options include:
- DC cardioversion [A]
- flecainide [A]
- ibutilide [A] 0.01 mg/kg to a maximum of 1 mg over 10 minutes
- amiodarone [A]
- procainamide [A] bolus of 10 mg per kg at a rate of 100 mg per minute

- propafenone [A] 150 mg orally three times a day (reduce dose if < 70 kg)
- quinidine 200 mg and verapamil 80 mg three times a day. [A]

DC cardioversion
- Patients with acute onset AF or flutter can be cardioverted immediately, [D] but should be started on heparin followed by a month of warfarin. [D]
- In cases of uncertain duration, anticoagulate your patient for a month before and after cardioversion. [C]
- Consider giving an infusion of ibutilide (0.01 mg/kg over 10 minutes) before cardioversion. [A]
- Check your patient has: [D]
  - INR > 2.0
  - K > 4.0 mmol/l
- Arrange for a general anaesthetic for your patient, and ensure your patient is starved for at least 6 hours. [A]
- Cardiovert starting at 100 J; followed by 100 J, 200 J, 300 J, 360 J. [D]

Flecainide
Contraindicated with ischaemic heart disease. [A]
- Intravenous – give 2 mg/kg (to a maximum of 150 mg) over 30 minutes.
- Oral – give 200 mg twice daily, reducing after 3 to 5 days to 50 mg daily.

Amiodarone
Loading dose:
- Intravenous:
  - Preferably via a central line.
  - Give 300 mg (5 mg/kg) in 250 ml 5.0% glucose over 1 hour, followed by 900 mg over 24 hours.
- Oral:
  - Give 200 mg every 8 hours for one week, then 200 mg every 12 hours for one week, then start maintenance therapy.

Maintenance dose:
- Patients should be given a total loading dose of 4200 mg before starting on maintenance therapy. [D]
- Give 100 to 200 mg daily.

Chronic atrial fibrillation

Control the ventricular rate [A] using digoxin [D], calcium-channel blockers or beta-blockers.

Consider conversion to sinus rhythm [A] using:
- DC cardioversion, [C] followed by amiodarone. [B]

Note
- Cardioversion is less likely to be successful if patients:
  - have had AF for 3 months or more [A]
  - have severe heart failure [A]
  - are old [A]
  - have rheumatic heart disease. [A]
- Warn patients that cardioversion may need to be repeated several times. [A]

Amiodarone
Loading dose:
- Intravenous:
  - Preferably via a central line.
  - Give 300 mg (5 mg/kg) in 250 ml 5.0% glucose over 1 hour, followed by 900 mg over 24 hours.
- Oral:
  - Give 200 mg every 8 hours for 1 week, then 200 mg every 12 hours for 1 week, then start maintenance therapy.

Maintenance dose:
- Patients should be given a total loading dose of 4200 mg before starting on maintenance therapy. [D]
- Give 100 to 200 mg daily.

Alternatives to amiodarone include:
- flecainide [B]
- disopyramide. [A]

Flecainide
Contraindicated with ischaemic heart disease. [A]
- Intravenous – give 2 mg/kg (to a maximum of 150 mg) over 30 minutes.
- Oral – give 200 mg twice daily, reducing after 3 to 5 days to 50 mg daily.

Disopyramide
Intravenous.
- Give 2 mg/kg (to a maximum of 150 mg) over 5 minutes.
- Followed by one of:
  - 400 μg/kg/hour i.v. – maximum 300 mg in first hour, and 800 mg daily.
  - 200 mg orally immediately, then 200 mg every 8 hours for 24 hours.

Consider pharmacological cardioversion if your patient is unsuitable for DC cardioversion [D] using one of:
- amiodarone [A]
- propafenone [A] 150 mg orally three times a day (reduce dose if < 70 kg).

For patients with symptomatic chronic AF resistant to medication, consider:
- radiofrequency AV node modulation [A]
- atriotomy. [C]

REVIEW

Anticoagulate patients who remain in or are at risk of relapsing back into atrial fibrillation. [A]
- Give warfarin [A] to patients with one or more other risk factors for stroke. [A]
- Give aspirin [A] 75 mg daily [A] to patients: [A]
  - at low risk of stroke (< 1% per year)
  - at high risk for a major bleed
  - who particularly dislike the thought of taking warfarin.

Warfarin
- Aim for INR 2.0 to 3.0. [B]
- See Chapter 19 for more details on warfarin therapy.

Atrial fibrillation and the risk of stroke

Age	No other risk factors for stroke	1 + other risk factors
< 65	1%	5%
65 to 75	4%	6%
> 75	4%	8%

Risk of bleeding on warfarin [A]
Score one point for each risk factor:
- Aged 65 or more.
- History of stroke.
- History of gastrointestinal bleeding.
- Any of recent myocardial infarction, haematocrit < 30%, Cr > 133 μmol/L or diabetes mellitus.

Score	Risk of major bleeding at 4 years
3 or 4	53%
1 or 2	12%
0	3%

Paroxysmal atrial fibrillation

Consider long-term anti-arrhythmic therapy in symptomatic cases. [D]
Start medication in hospital. [C]

Consider using one of:
- amiodarone [A]
- flecainide – at least 100 mg twice daily [A]
- propafenone [A] 300 mg orally twice daily [A]
- sotalol – at least 120 mg twice daily. [A]

Note
There is no clear benefit from long-term digoxin with paroxysmal AF. [D]

For patients with intolerable paroxysmal AF resistant to anti-arrhythmic medication, consider:
- Ablation of the AV node and insertion of a DDDR permanent pacemaker. [A]
- An implantable atrial defibrillator. [C]

Outcomes
- Half of patients with acute AF revert spontaneously to sinus rhythm within 18 hours. [A]
- Up to half of patients with paroxysmal AF will have a recurrent symptomatic episode within a year.
- Few patients with chronic AF remain in sinus rhythm following one DC cardioversion. [A]

8
BRADYARRHYTHMIAS

SYMPTOMS AND SIGNS

Look for symptomatic bradycardia: [C]
- heart failure – fatigue, dyspnoea and oedema
- syncope or pre-syncope
- angina
- hypotension.

Common causes of bradyarrhythmias [B,D]
- myocardial infarction
- sick sinus syndrome (symptomatic bradycardia < 50 beats per minute or symptomatic PRS pauses > 2 seconds)
- drugs
- hypothermia
- hypothyroidism
- fitness.

INVESTIGATIONS

- Temperature. [C]
- Urea and electrolytes. [D]
- Cardiac enzymes. [B]
- Thyroid function tests. [C]
- ECG. [A]

THERAPY

Stop any medication potentially causing bradycardia, e.g. beta-blockers, digoxin, diltiazem. [D]

Give atropine 1 mg to a maximum of 3 mg i.v. [C] to symptomatic patients. [D]

Set up temporary pacing for patients:
- who remain symptomatic [A]
- with episodes of ventricular standstill [A]
- with an anterior myocardial infarction with Mobitz II or 3rd degree heart block. [D]

Heart block
Consider giving an infusion of potassium, glucose and insulin in 2nd or 3rd degree heart block if pacing is not available. [C]

Arrange for a permanent pacemaker for patients with:

- sick sinus syndrome [A]
- carotid sinus syndrome [A]
- ventricular standstill [A]
- Mobitz II or 3rd degree heart block. [A]

9
CARBON MONOXIDE POISONING

SYMPTOMS AND SIGNS

Ask about:
- symptoms of carbon monoxide poisoning: [C]
  - headache
  - dizziness
  - nausea, vomiting, diarrhoea
  - visual disturbances, focal neurological signs, seizures
  - loss of consciousness.

- exposure to carbon monoxide: [D]
  - vehicle exhaust fumes in a contained environment
  - a combustion stove with a non-functioning exhaust system
  - fire exposure in a contained environment.

> **Think about CO poisoning in:** [C]
> - victims of accidental or intentional CO exposure
> - patients with non-specific symptoms (e.g. headaches, nausea)
> - unconscious patients without a clear cause.

INVESTIGATIONS

- Arterial blood gas. [D] N.B. Do not use pulse oximetry alone – it can be deceptively reassuring.
- Carboxyhaemoglobin level (arterial or venous sample). [C]
- ECG monitoring. [C]
- Chest X-ray. [C]

> **Abnormal carboxyhaemoglobin levels** [C]
> - Smokers > 10%.
> - Non-smokers > 5%.

THERAPY

- Assess airway, breathing, circulation. [D]
- 100% oxygen by rebreather mask for 6 hours and repeat for 100 minutes for at least 3 days (with simple high-flow oxygen in between). [A]

Hyperbaric oxygen

Avoid using hyperbaric oxygen [A] – it is not clearly any better than normobaric oxygen, and can cause complications (ear barotrauma, oxygen toxicity, severe claustrophobia).

Outcomes

- Early neurological impairment is common, but usually settles within a month. [B]
- Few patients die. [C]

Expires July 2005   Guideline: Joel Ray, Chris Ball
                        CATs: Joel Ray, Chris Ball, Clare Wotton

10
CARDIAC ARREST

PREPARATION

- Go on a life support course before joining a cardiac arrest team. [A]
- Ask patients on admission to hospital whether they want cardiopulmonary resuscitation [A] and educate them about the chances of survival. [C]

Note
Neither clinicians [C] nor clinical prediction rules [A] accurately predict which patients will survive a hospital cardiac arrest based on information available in the first 24 hours.

IMMEDIATE MANAGEMENT

Run to the arrest. [A]

Start basic life support: [A]

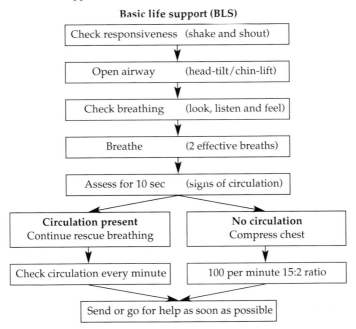

Basic life support (BLS)

Check responsiveness (shake and shout)
↓
Open airway (head-tilt/chin-lift)
↓
Check breathing (look, listen and feel)
↓
Breathe (2 effective breaths)
↓
Assess for 10 sec (signs of circulation)
↓
Circulation present — Continue rescue breathing | **No circulation** — Compress chest
↓
Check circulation every minute | 100 per minute 15:2 ratio
↓
Send or go for help as soon as possible

If possible, perform:
- active compression–decompression CPR using a cardiopump [B]
- or interposed abdominal counterpulsation: compression over the umbilicus to co-ordinate with early relaxation of chest compression (rate 80 to 100 per minute). [A]

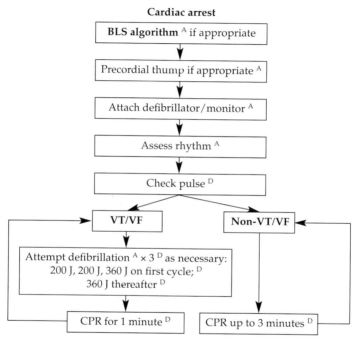

Cardiac arrest

BLS algorithm [A] if appropriate

↓

Precordial thump if appropriate [A]

↓

Attach defibrillator/monitor [A]

↓

Assess rhythm [A]

↓

Check pulse [D]

VT/VF   **Non-VT/VF**

Attempt defibrillation [A] × 3 [D] as necessary:
200 J, 200 J, 360 J on first cycle; [D]
360 J thereafter [D]

CPR for 1 minute [D]   CPR up to 3 minutes [D]

During CPR
- Check electrode/paddle positions and contacts. [A]
- Attempt to place, confirm and secure airway [A] and give oxygen. [A]
  - Insert a laryngeal mask if unfamiliar with endotracheal tubes. [B]
- Attempt and verify early i.v. access. [A]

Patients with VT/VF refractory to initial shocks:
- adrenaline [D] 1 mg [D] every 3 to 5 minutes [D] or
- vasopressin [A] 40 units i.v. single dose once only.

Patients with non-VT/VF rhythms:
- adrenaline [D] 1 mg [D] every 3 to 5 minutes. [D]

Note
None of these agents has been shown to have any effect on the number of patients leaving hospital alive.

Consider:
- buffers [D]
- antiarrhythmics: [D]
  - amiodarone [A] 150–300 mg i.v. over 1–2 min
  - lignocaine [B] 100 mg i.v. (5 ml of 2% solution) over 30 sec
  - magnesium 1 g if hypomagnesaemic [D]
  - procainamide 100 mg i.v. every 5 min to a maximum of 1 g if intermittent recurrent VT/VF [D]
- atropine [B] 3 mg i.v. or pacing [D]
- calcium chloride [B] 10 ml of 10%
- bretylium [B] 5 mg/kg i.v. bolus, followed by 10 mg/kg i.v. after 5 min if VT persists.

Search for and correct reversible causes. [A]

Think about potentially reversible causes
- hypoxia
- hypovolaemia
- hydrogen ion – acidosis
- hypo- or hyperkalaemia and other metabolic disorders
- hypothermia
- tension pneumothorax
- tamponade
- toxic/therapeutic disturbances
- thrombosis (coronary)
- thrombosis (pulmonary embolism).

Consider stopping the resuscitation if all the following are present: [A]
- > 10 minutes since CPR started
- initial rhythm not VT or VF
- arrest not witnessed.

INVESTIGATIONS

- Blood count. [D]
- U&E, creatinine. [D]
- 12-lead ECG.
- Arterial blood gas. [D]
- Chest X-ray. [D]

REVIEW

In survivors, watch out for post-arrest complications including: [B]
- rib fractures
- marrow emboli

- haemopericardium
- liver or spleen lacerations.

For patients who had a VT or VF arrest, consider:
- amiodarone [A]
- implantable defibrillators. [A]

Outcomes
- One in six patients are discharged alive. [B] Survival is worse with:
  - out-of-hospital cardiac arrests [B]
  - asystole or pulseless electrical activity [A]
  - increasing age. [B]
- Recovery is good in patients who survive to be discharged, but one in seven have another cardiac arrest within a year. [C]
- A quarter are dead within 5 years. [C]

11
CELLULITIS

SYMPTOMS AND SIGNS

Most cases of cellulitis are obvious. Look for: [C]
- pain or tenderness
- erythema
- increased warmth
- swelling
- temperature $\geq 37.7°C$
- regional lymphadenopathy.

Look for a possible cause: [B]
- a site of entry (e.g. leg ulcer, toe-web intertrigo, traumatic wound)
- lymphoedema, leg oedema or venous insufficiency
- obesity.

Ask about diabetes mellitus [A] and look for osteomyelitis if there is: [A]
- an ulcer > 2 cm^2
- bone exposed within an ulcer
- bone palpable with a sterile probe in an ulcer.

Think about other causes of hot swollen legs
- DVT
- Baker's cyst
- Necrotizing fasciitis.

DVT
If a DVT is possible, further investigations are required, e.g. ultrasound scanning.
See Chapter 16 for more details.

Baker's cyst
If a Baker's cyst is possible, look for: [B]
+ crepitus on flexing the knee
+ a history of arthritis
+ a positive ultrasound scan.

Remember – the presence of a Baker's cyst does not exclude a DVT.

Necrotizing fasciitis

Think about necrotizing fasciitis if there is: ^{C}

- crepitus
- sensation loss
- severe pain.

INVESTIGATIONS

■ Swab any skin breaks, wounds or ulcers. ^{C}

Consider:
■ a blood count ^{D}
■ glucose ^{D}
■ blood cultures. ^{D}

If osteomyelitis is a possibility, consider: ^{A}
+ ESR
+ a bone scan
± an MRI.

Note

X-rays are usually unhelpful at diagnosing osteomyelitis. ^{A}

If necrotizing fasciitis is a possibility, consider: ^{C}
± frozen biopsy
± an MRI.

THERAPY

- Give analgesia. ^{D}
- Give antibiotics ^{A} to cover *Staphylococcus* and *Streptococcus* – e.g. flucloxacillin 500 mg q.d.s. and benzylpencillin 600 mg q.d.s. for 7 days.
  - Admit patients with systemic signs of sepsis for intravenous antibiotics. ^{D}
- Urgent surgery is required for necrotizing fasciitis. ^{D}

Common infecting organisms

- *Staphylococcus* with *Streptococcus*
- *Staphylococcus* alone
- *Streptococcus* alone
- *Klebsiella*
- others (including *Pseudomonas*).

REVIEW

Review patients who are treated as outpatients, since some are not cured. [C]

Preventing cellulitis
- Clean wounds with povidone-iodine. [B]
- Give prophlyactic antibiotics for:
  - dog bites [A]
  - human bites [A] – remember to cover anaerobes!

Expires July 2004 Guideline John Epling, Chris Ball
CATs: John Epling, Chris Ball

12
CHEST PAIN

SYMPTOMS AND SIGNS

Ask about:
- the pain, specifically:
    - its position, [B] looking for:
        + retrosternal or left arm pain [B] (if MI suspected)
        + pain migration [C] (if aortic dissection suspected)

    - its duration, [A] looking for:
        + chest pain which started ≥ 48 hours ago [A] (if MI suspected)
        + constant pain [B] (if MI suspected)

    - its nature, [A] looking for:
        + pressure [A] (if MI or UA suspected)
        − sharp or stabbing pain [A] (if MI or UA suspected)
        − pleuritic pain [A] (its presence makes a PE more likely and MI or UA unlikely)
        − positional pain [A] (if MI or UA suspected)

    + any similarity to previous infarcts or angina attacks [A]

    - any exacerbating or relieving factors, [B] particularly:
        + pain brought on by exertion
        + pain relieved by nitrates or rest

- associated symptoms:
    - nausea or vomiting [B] (if MI suspected)
    - sweating [B] (if MI suspected)
    - haemoptysis [A] (if PE suspected)
    - dyspnoea or worsening of chronic dyspnoea [A] (if PE suspected)

- a history of:
    + angina or MI [A] (if MI or UA suspected)
    + hypertension [B] (if aortic dissection suspected)
    + asthma [A]
    + dementia [A] (if pneumonia suspected)
    + immunosuppression [A] (if pneumonia suspected)
    + Marfan syndrome [A] (if aortic dissection suspected)

- cardiovascular risk factors:
    - hypertension [A]
    - smoking [B]
    - diabetes mellitus [A]
    - elevated total cholesterol or triglycerides [A]

- a parental history of angina or MI before the age of 60 [A] (if MI suspected)

- risk factors for venous thromboembolism:
  - recent immobilization: [A]
    - paralysis of a leg [A]
    - surgery or a fracture of the leg with immobilization within the last 12 weeks [A]
    - recently bedridden for > 3 days within the last 4 weeks [A]
  - previous venous thromboembolism (objective diagnosis) [A]
  - a strong family history of DVT or PE:
    - 2 or more family members with objectively-proven events [A]
    - a first-degree relative with hereditary thrombophilia [A]
  - active cancer (on-going treatment, diagnosed within last 6 months or having palliative care) [a]
  - post-partum. [A]

Common causes of chest pain include: [C]
- myocardial infarction
- unstable angina
- pulmonary embolism
- chest infection
- musculoskeletal pain
- pericarditis.

Rarer causes include: [D]
- aortic dissection
- oesophageal spasm
- oesophageal rupture
- abdominal pain
  - gallstones
  - gastritis
- herpes zoster.

Think about causes of pleuritic chest pain [A]
- pulmonary embolism
- viral
- pneumonia
- chest wall trauma
- cancer.

Look for:
- general:
  - fever [A] (if pneumonia suspected)
  - respiratory rate > 30 per minute [A] (if pneumonia suspected)

- tachycardia [A] (if pneumonia suspected)
- sweating [B] (if MI suspected)

- cardiovascular system:
  - hypertension [C] or hypotension [B] (if aortic dissection suspected)
  + absent or reduced pulses [C] (if aortic dissection suspected)
  + a third heart sound [B] (if MI suspected)
  − chest pain that is reproduced on palpation [A] (if MI or UA suspected)

- respiratory system:
  - a cough [A] (if pneumonia suspected)
  - arterial oxygen saturation < 92% when breathing room air that corrects with 40% O_2 (if PE suspected)
  + asymmetric respiration [A] (if pneumonia suspected)
  + chest dullness on percussion [A] (if pneumonia suspected)
  + decreased breath sounds [A] (if pneumonia suspected)
  + bronchial breathing [A] (if pneumonia suspected)
  + crackles [A] (if pneumonia suspected)
  + aegophony [A] (if pneumonia suspected)
  - pleural rub [A] (if PE suspected)

- neurological system:
  - evidence of a stroke or paralysis [B] (if aortic dissection suspected).

Estimate your patient's risk of significant coronary artery disease (> 50% coronary artery stenosis in at least one major artery – see Tables 6.1 and 6.2) using age [A] and the following symptoms: [B]
+ retrosternal chest pain
+ pain brought on by exertion
+ pain relieved in < 10 minutes by rest or GTN.

INVESTIGATIONS

- Blood count. [B]
- U&E, creatinine. [D]
- Glucose. [D]
- Serial cardiac enzymes (when diagnosing MI):
  ± CK-MB over 24 hours [C]
  ± troponin T [C]
  ± creatine kinase [B] over 48 hours with:
    + lactate dehydrogenase. [A]
- Lipid levels. [A]
- Arterial blood gas if dyspnoeic. [D]
± 12-lead ECG, [A] followed by serial ECGs. [B]
- Chest X-ray. [A]

Cardiac enzymes
- An early CK-MB rise diagnoses a myocardial infarction and normal levels at 20 hours rule it out. ^C
- A normal troponin T or troponin I at 20 hours makes an infarct unlikely. ^C
- Elevated creatine kinase levels ^B or an elevated myoglobin ^C diagnoses an infarct.
- CK, AST or LDH taken on presentation cannot safely diagnose or exclude an infarct. ^A

ECG
- Look for features suggesting cardiac ischaemia:
  - any ST elevation in 2 or more leads ^A
  - any ST depression ^B
  - any Q waves ^A
  - any T wave inversion ^B
  - any conduction defect. ^B
- These are more significant if present in 2 or more leads, or not known to be old.
- A normal ECG makes life-threatening complications unlikely. ^C

Chest X-ray
- Look for:
  - a lobar infiltrate ^C (if pneumonia suspected)
  - widening of the aorta (particularly the knob) or mediastinum ^B (if aortic dissection suspected)
  - pleural effusion ^B (if aortic dissection suspected)
  - tracheal shift ^B (if aortic dissection suspected)

Patients at low risk for a myocardial infarction can be assessed in a rapid evaluation unit by: ^D
- CK-MB at 0, 4, 8, 12 hours
- serial 12-lead ECGs
- clinical assessment at 0, 6, 12 hours
- exercise ECG: if all the above are negative.

Need for coronary care unit admission
Use the clinical prediction rule given in Table 6.3 to help you determine whether your patient needs admission to a coronary care unit. ^A

Table 12.1 Risk of myocardial infarction
Continue down the first column until you match a clinical feature with one of
your patient's. Then go across to the second column if applicable and continue
until another matching clinical feature is found, and then read the risk in the
third column.

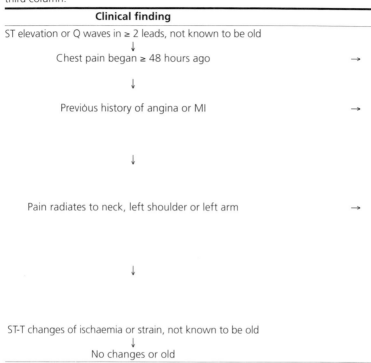

Clinical finding
ST elevation or Q waves in ≥ 2 leads, not known to be old
↓
Chest pain began ≥ 48 hours ago →
↓
Previous history of angina or MI →
↓
Pain radiates to neck, left shoulder or left arm →
↓
ST-T changes of ischaemia or strain, not known to be old
↓
No changes or old

Use the above clinical prediction rule (Table 12.1) to rank your patient for
risk of a myocardial infarction. [A]

Stress testing
Perform stress testing before discharge or as an outpatient [D] using any
of:

± a symptom-limited [C] exercise tolerance test [A]
± myocardial perfusion scanning [A] looking for a reversible perfusion
   defect [B]

	Risk of MI
	75%
ST-T changes of ischaemia or strain, not known to be old	20%
↓ No changes or old	2%
ST-T changes of ischaemia or strain, not known to be old	25%
↓ Longest pain episode < 1 hour	4%
↓ Pain worse than prior angina or the same as a prior MI	10%
↓ Pain not as bad	1%
Aged < 40	2%
↓ Chest pain reproduced by palpation	1%
↓ Pain radiates to back, abdomen or legs	8%
↓ Chest pain stabbing	2%
↓ Chest pain not stabbing	20%
	25%
	2%

± exercise SPECT (single photon emission CT) [A]
± exercise echocardiography. [A]

Refer all patients for coronary angiography (followed by PTCA or CABG as required) if they develop:
- spontaneous angina occurring > 36 hours after admission [A]
- prolonged angina with an ischaemic ECG
- abnormal stress testing [A]
- moderate to severe angina after hospital discharge despite maximal anti-ischaemic therapy. [A]

Exercise ECG

Look for: [B]

- horizontal or down-sloping ST slope and 1 mm or more of depression in any lead [B]
- angina during the test
- limited exercise duration
- impaired systolic blood pressure changes
- signs of poor ventricular function: ejection fraction < 40%.

Use the following clinical prediction rule to rank your patient for risk of dying. [A]

Total score = D – (5 × M) – (4 × T)

where   D = duration of exercise in minutes
M = maximal ST-segment deviation during or after exercise in mm
T = treadmill angina index (see Table 6.4).

Interpretation of the total score is shown in Table 6.5.

Consider performing oesophageal tests (manometry) [C] after coronary artery disease has been excluded, but use the results with caution, since they may not indicate the true course.

THERAPY

See the relevant chapter for more information on the management of:
- aortic dissection (Ch. 4)
- bradyarrhythmias (Ch. 8)
- myocardial infarction (Ch. 30)
- community-acquired pneumonia (Ch. 32)
- pulmonary embolism (Ch. 34)
- tachycardias (Ch. 40)
- unstable angina (Ch. 6).

Consider trying the following for patients with chest pain who continue to have symptoms, but have had cardiac disease excluded:
- a proton-pump inhibitor [A]
- imipramine [A]
- cognitive–behavioural therapy. [A]

Note
- Be cautious about discharging patients even with a low risk of a myocardial infarction. [B]
- One in five patients with acute chest pain is dead within 3 years. [A]

Expires July 2003   Guideline: Chris Ball
CATs: Chris Ball, Clare Wotton, Nick Shenker

13
DECOMPENSATED CHRONIC LIVER FAILURE

SYMPTOMS AND SIGNS

Ask about:
+ alcohol intake [B]
+ known hepatitis [A]
■ previous variceal bleeding [D] and recent GI haemorrhage [A]
■ previous episodes of spontaneous bacterial peritonitis [A]
+ previous ascites [A]
− recent ankle swelling [A] (if ascites suspected)
± increasing girth [A]
+ recent weight gain. [A]

Look for:
+ facial telangiectasia [A]
+ spider naevi [A]
+ abdominal wall veins [A]
+ white nails [A]
+ obesity [A]
+ peripheral oedema. [A]

Risk of cirrhosis [B]
High (> 80%) if:
• all 6 signs present and peripheral oedema
• ≥ 4 signs if no peripheral oedema
• ≥ 3 signs if facial telangiectasia and no peripheral oedema.

Moderate if:
• any other combination.

Low (< 20%) if:
• no facial telangiectasia and ≤ 2 other signs.

Look for other features of cirrhosis:
+ jaundice [A]
+ palmar erythema [A]
+ gynaecomastia in men [A]
+ sparse axillary or pubic hair [A]
+ testicular atrophy [A]
■ cachexia [B]
+ hepatomegaly. [A]

> **Causes of cirrhosis include:** C
> - alcohol
> - cryptogenic
> - hepatitis B or C
> - haemachromatosis.

Look for complications, including:

+ signs of encephalopathy. A

> **Hepatic encephalopathy** D
>
> | Grade | Signs |
> |-------|-------|
> | 1 | Confused; altered mood or behaviour |
> | 2 | Drowsy with inappropriate behaviour |
> | 3 | Stupor with inarticulate speech |
> | | Rousable and can obey simple commands |
> | 4 | Coma |
> | | Unrousable |

- ascites – look for: A
  - bulging flanks
  - ± peripheral oedema
  - ± a fluid wave
  - + shifting dullness and flank dullness
- evidence of sepsis C

> **Think about spontaneous bacterial peritonitis with:** D
> - temperature up or down, *and* diarrhoea
> - abdominal pain
> - encephalopathy.

- evidence of coagulopathy, D e.g. bruising, petechiae
- evidence of acute bleeding B
  + supine tachycardia
  + supine hypotension (systolic blood presure < 95 mmHg)
  + postural pulse increase of > 30 beats/min or severe dizziness on sitting upright, or standing.

> **Note**
> Postural hypotension does not usefully diagnose acute blood loss. B

See Chapter 41 for more details.

INVESTIGATIONS

- Blood count. [D]
- Clotting. [A]
- U&E, creatinine. [A]
- Liver function tests. [A]
- Glucose. [D]
- Blood cultures. [D]
- Arterial blood gases. [D]
- Chest X-ray. [D]

Watch out for:
- low platelet counts [D]
- abnormal clotting [D]
- hyponatraemia [D]
- hypoglycaemia [A]
- hypoalbuminaemia [D]
- hepatorenal syndrome – renal dysfunction is common. [C]

Consider:
- hepatitis serology [A]
- toxicology screen including paracetamol [D]
- an abdominal ultrasound [D]
- an ascitic tap, particularly [D] with:
    - any unexplained ascites
    - explained ascites, when it first appears
    - any patient with liver disease and suspected bacterial peritonitis
- liver biopsy for newly diagnosed cases [D]
- upper GI endoscopy.

Ascitic tap
Order: [D]
- white cell count and differential. Look for > 250 neutrophils/μl [C] – this diagnoses spontaneous bacterial peritonitis
- microscopy, culture and sensitivities [A]
- cytology [A]
- amylase [D]
- protein. [A]

Consider:
- inserting a urinary catheter to monitor urine output [D]
- an echocardiogram [D]
- daily weights. [D]

THERAPY

Correct: [D]
- hypoxia
- hypotension
- hypoglycaemia
- hypokalaemia.

Give thiamine 100 mg [D] i.v. [C] to alcoholics or malnourished patients. [D]

Ascites
- Perform paracentesis, [A] drawing off 4 to 6 litres per day, followed by 20% salt-poor albumin [A] or long-acting colloids (e.g. hydroxyethyl starch). [A]
- Give spironolactone [A] 300 mg daily.

Encephalopathy
Consider:
- lactulose 20 ml 4 times a day [A] (rectally or via nasogastric tube if required [D])
- neomycin 1 g orally every 4 hours [A]
- a flumazenil infusion. [A]

Spontaneous bacterial peritonitis
- Give antibiotics [A] i.v. [D] e.g. cefotaxime 2 g every 6 hours [A] with albumin [A] (1.5 g/kg over 6 hours, followed by 1 g/kg 2 days later).

Varices
- Arrange for endoscopic ligation [B] or sclerotherapy [A] within 6 hours. [B]
- Give octreotide or somatostatin.

Somatostatin
Somatostatin 6 mg in 500 ml 0.9% saline i.v. over 24 hours for 5 days.

Octreotide
- Give a bolus of octreotide 50 μg i.v. followed by
- Octreotide 500 μg in 50 ml 0.9% saline at 50 μg per hour (i.e. 5 ml/h).

See Chapter 41 for more details.

Consider:
- balloon tamponade [a] for patients who do not stop bleeding [d]
- transjugular intrahepatic portosystemic shunts (TIPPS). [D]

REVIEW

Monitor: [D]
- clotting
- electrolytes
- glucose
- liver function tests.

Perform daily weights. [D]

Spontaneous bacterial peritonitis
On recovery, prescribe prophylactic antibiotics, e.g. norfloxacin 40 mg daily [A] or trimethoprim-sulfamethoxazole double-strength tablets 5 times a week. [B]

Varices
- Arrange for endoscopic ligation [A] or sclerotherapy [A] until varices are obliterated.
- Give beta-blockers [A] (e.g. propranolol MR 80 mg daily) or isosorbide mononitrate MR [A] 60 mg daily.
- Consider giving mannitol whole-gut irrigation following a variceal bleed to reduce encephalopathy. [A]

Mannitol whole-gut irrigation
Run a 5-litre solution containing 40 g/L mannitol via nasogastric tube over 2.5 hours.

Risk of dying
Refer to Table 13.1.

Table 13.1   Risk of dying

Prognostic factor [A]	Points
Age ≥ 65	1
Cognitive dysfunction:	
• GCS 10 to 14 (see Table 15.1)	1
• GCS < 10 (see Table 15.1)	2
Renal insufficiency:	
• creatinine 88 to 176 μmol/L	1
• creatinine > 176 μmol/L	2
Prothrombin time ≥ 16 seconds	1
Mechanical ventilation or hypoxia (pO_2 < 60 mmHg)	1

Score [A]	Risk of death at 6 months
≥ 4	High (80%)
2 to 3	Moderate (60%)
≤1	Low (30%)

Outcomes
- One in four patients with ascites develops spontaneous bacterial peritonitis within a year [A] – over half die. [A] It recurs in half of survivors. [A]
- One in five develops bleeding from oesophageal varices within 3 years. [A]
- One in four with decompensated cirrhosis dies in hospital, and half are dead within 6 months. [A]

14
EXACERBATION OF CHRONIC OBSTRUCTIVE PULMONARY DISEASE

SYMPTOMS AND SIGNS

Ask about:
+ a history of COPD [A]
+ smoking [A] and how much for how long [A]
■ number of previous exacerbations [B] and the need for steroids or ventilation [D]
+ cough [A]
+ wheezing [A]
+ exertional dyspnoea [A]
+ sputum production [A] and any recent increase in quantity or purulence. [D]

> **Think about other causes of dypsnoea** [B]
> * asthma
> * heart failure
> * arrhythmia
> * infection
> * interstitial lung disease
> * anaemia
> * pulmonary embolism
> * pneumothorax. [D]

Look for:
■ tachypnoea [D]
■ cyanosis [D]
■ signs of CO_2 retention (warm peripheries, bounding pulse, tachycardia, flap) [D]
+ a reduced laryngeal height (≤ 4 cm) [A]
+ a barrel chest [A]
+ hyperresonance [A]
+ decreased cardiac dullness. [A]

Listen for:
+ decreased breath sounds
+ wheezing or crackles [B]
+ a prolonged expiratory time.

> **Note** [B]
> COPD can be confidently diagnosed if all the following are present:
> * a self-reported history of COPD
> * smoking > 40 pack-years

- aged 45 or more
- maximum laryngeal height ≤ 4 cm.

Forced expiratory time [A]
Measure the time expiratory sounds are audible over the sternum during forced expiration. COPD is more likely if > 9 sec.

INVESTIGATIONS

- Blood count. [D]
- U&E, creatinine. [D]
- Cardiac enzymes. [D]
- Blood culture if infection suspected. [D]
- Sputum culture if infection suspected. [D]
- Arterial blood gases [B] under local anaesthetic. [A]
- ECG. [A]
- Chest X-ray in all patients. [A]
- Peak expiratory flow-rate. [A]

Arterial blood gases
One in five patients has CO_2 retention. [B]

ECG changes
Look for: [A]
+ right heart failure
+ ischaemic heart disease.

Chest X-ray
Note: clinical features do not usefully predict normal films.

Consider:
- spirometry [A] when better.

THERAPY

- Give oxygen if hypoxic [A] via mask or nasal cannula. [D] Use low concentrations to prevent CO_2 narcosis and monitor pCO_2 levels. [A]

Aim to keep: [D]
- $pCO_2 < 8.0$ kPa
- $pO_2 > 6.5$ kPa
with a normal pH (7.35 to 7.45).
If this is not possible, arrange for non-invasive ventilation. [A]

- Salbutamol 5 mg [D] nebulizers if wheezy.
- Antibiotics. [A]

Follow local prescribing guidelines. [D]
Reasonable choices include:
- a second-generation cephalosporin, [A] e.g. cephalexin 500 mg t.d.s.
- co-amoxiclav [A] 625 mg t.d.s.
- a quinolone, [A] e.g. ciprofloxacin 400 mg b.d.
- a macrolide, [A] e.g. erythromycin 500 mg q.d.s.

Consider:
- systemic steroids, [A] e.g. oral prednisolone 30 mg daily
- aminophylline [A] in severe cases. [D]

Aminophylline
- Add 250 mg to 500 ml of 0.9% saline.
- Give a loading dose of 5.6 mg/kg over 20 min (not if patient has received aminophylline or oral theophylline in last 24 hours), followed by continuous infusion 0.9 mg/kg per hour (0.45 ml/kg per hour).
- Monitor theophylline levels [A] daily (therapeutic range 10–20 mg/L).
- Watch for features of toxicity (e.g. nausea, vomiting, arrhythmias).

For patients with respiratory failure (worsening hypoxia or hypercapnia, exhaustion or confusion), consider non-invasive ventilation, [A] e.g. CPAP.

REVIEW

- Swap patients to inhalers as symptoms improve. [D]
- Gradually reduce the steroid dose over the next few weeks (e.g. reduce by 5 mg every 4 days until stopped).

- Advise your patient to stop smoking. [A]
- Advise your patient to receive influenza [B] and pneumococcal vaccination. [A]

Offer:
- respiratory rehabilitation [A]
- continuous home oxygen to patients with severe hypoxia (pO_2 < 7.5 kPa or < 8.0 kPa with oedema). [A]

Outcomes
- One in twelve dies in hospital. [B]
- Further exacerbations and readmissions are common, particularly with bronchitis, daily wheeze, or frequent exacerbations in the past. [B]
- One in four dies within 3 years. [B] The risk is increased with worsening symptoms, heart failure, ischaemic heart disease or chronic renal failure. [A]

Expires July 2003 Guideline: Chris Ball
CATs: Chris Ball, Clare Wotton, Bob Phillips

15
COMA

IMMEDIATE MANAGEMENT

- Get help.
- Assess the airway and breathing:
  - clear the airway [A] and stabilize the cervical spine if there is a history of head or neck trauma [A]
  - ventilate with a bag-valve-mask and 100% oxygen [A]
  - consider intubation. [D]
- Assess the circulation: [D]
  - correct any hypovolaemia or arrhythmias [D]
  - obtain large bore i.v. access and consider central venous pressure monitoring. [D]
- Look for evidence of hypoglycaemia: [C]
  - measure glucose rapidly using reagent strips [A] or capillary blood glucose in triage [A]
  - measure blood glucose [A]
  - if you believe hypoglycaemia is present, try a test dose of 50% glucose i.v. [A]

> **Note**
> Remember patients with diabetes may experience hypoglycaemia at 'normoglycaemic' levels. [D]

- Give thiamine 100 mg i.v. [D] to alcoholics or malnourished patients. [D]
- Look for status epilepticus: [C]
  - if present give lorazepam 0.1 mg/kg at 2 mg/min.

> **Note**
> Signs of fitting may be subtle – look for twitching of extremities, mouth and eyes. [C]

- Correct hypothermia.
- Assess the level of consciousness using the Glasgow Coma Scale (Table 15.1). [A]

Table 15.1 Glasgow Coma Scale (GCS)

Eye opening	Score
Spontaneous	4
On verbal command	3
To pain	2
No response	1

Table 15.1 (*Continued*)

Eye opening	Score
Motor response	
Correct response to 'show me 2 fingers'	6
Localizes pain and tries to stop it	5
Withdraws from painful stimuli to fingernail	4
Abnormal flexor response of forearms, wrists and fingers	3
Abnormal extensor response of arms and legs	2
No response	1
Verbal response to question 'what year is this?'	
Correct year	5
Wrong year	4
Words but no year	3
Incomprehensible sounds	2
No response	1

Minimum score: 3
Maximum score: 15

- Treat any underlying cause. [A]

> **Common causes include:** [C]
> - overdose
> - trauma
> - shock
> - cardiac arrest
> - stroke or cerebral haemorrhage
> - hepatic encephalopathy
> - hypoglycaemia.
>
> **Rare but important causes include:** [D]
> - infection
> - brain tumour
> - uraemia and other metabolic disorders
> - psychogenic.

Traumatic brain injury
- Cool the patient down. [A]

> **Note**
> There is no clear benefit from:
> - hyperventilation [D]
> - steroids [D]
> - mannitol [D]
> - hypertonic saline. [D]

SIGNS AND SYMPTOMS

Ask ambulance crews, family, friends and clinicians who know the patient about:
- known allergies [D]
- recent symptoms [D]
- recent head injury [D]
- speed of onset of coma [D]
- previous episodes of coma [D]
- medical history [D]
- drug use. [D]

If you suspect an opiate overdose, ask about: [B]
- ± drug paraphernalia where the patient was found
- ± history of i.v. drug use from bystanders.

Look for evidence of:
- head injury [D]
- drug overdose [D]
- uraemia or other metabolic derangement [D]
- malignancy [C]
- stroke or cerebral haemorrhage [C]
- infection (brain, meninges, sepsis) [C]
- hypertension. [C]

If you suspect an opiate overdose, look for: [B]
- ± a reduced respiratory rate
- ± pinpoint pupils
- ± needle track marks on skin.

Look for raised intracranial pressure by assessing the fundi. Look for:
- papilloedema [D]
- ± absence of retinal vein pulsation [C]
- changes associated with diabetes or hypertension. [D]

Assess brainstem function: [D]
- pupillary response
- corneal reflex
- facial response to pain
- oculocephalic reflex (if no cervical spine trauma)
- oculovestibular reflex (if unruptured tympanic membrane)
- cough or gag reflex.

Brainstem function
- Oculocephalic reflex (doll's eye movement): rotate head from side to side; if the brainstem is intact, the eyes will move conjugately in the opposite direction from head rotation.
- Oculovestibular reflex: inject 200 ml of iced water into one ear. A normal response is the slow-phase of nystagmus towards the irrigated ear.

INVESTIGATIONS

- Capillary glucose. D
- Arterial blood gases. D
- Blood count. C
- Urea and electrolytes, creatinine. C
- Glucose. C
- Calcium. D
- ECG. D
- Chest X-ray. D
- CT head. D

Consider:
- serum and urine drugs screen if an overdose is suspected D
- blood culture if there is evidence of infection D
- cervical spine X-rays if trauma D
- lumbar puncture if signs of raised intracranial pressure are absent on CT head, and infection or intracranial haemorrhage is suspected. D

Suspected overdose
- Give flumazenil A 400 µg i.v. D
- Give naloxone B 400 µg i.m. followed by 400 µg i.v. D

REVIEW

Remember the continuing care of the unconscious patient, including:
- DVT prophylaxis A
- pressure sore prevention D
- corneal protection D
- nutrition. D

Monitor patients neurologically (Glasgow Coma Scale and pupil reaction). A

Consider arranging an EEG if there is no improvement in the level of consciousness after 1 week. B

More information can be found in the following chapters:
- diabetic ketoacidosis (Ch. 18)
- hypercalcaemia (Ch. 22)
- hypertensive crisis (Ch. 24)
- acute hypoglycaemia (Ch. 25)
- meningitis (Ch. 29)
- stroke (Ch. 38).

Expires July 2003   Guideline: Will Whiteley, Chris Ball
CATs: Will Whiteley, Chris Ball, Clare Wotton

16
DEEP VEIN THROMBOSIS

SYMPTOMS AND SIGNS

Use the following clinical prediction rule to work out your patient's risk of a deep vein thrombosis. [A] For patients with symptoms in both legs, use the more symptomatic leg.

> **Note**
> DVT cannot be safely diagnosed or excluded on history and physical examination alone. Imaging studies are necessary. [A]

Ask about	Score
Active cancer (on-going treatment, diagnosed within last 6 months or having palliative care)	+1
Paralysis, paresis or plaster immobilization of a leg	+1
Recently bedridden for > 3 days or major surgery within the last 4 weeks	+1

Look for	Score
Localized tenderness over distribution of the deep veins	+1
Entire leg swollen	+1
Calf circumference 10 cm below tibial tuberosity more than 3 cm greater than the other calf	+1
Pitting oedema only in the symptomatic leg	+1
Collateral dilated (but not varicose) veins	+1
An alternative diagnosis as likely as or more likely than DVT	−2

Score	Risk of DVT
3 or more	75%
1 to 2	17%
0 or less	3%

> **Think about other causes of unilateral leg swelling** [A]
> Common causes include:
> - cellulitis
> - muscle injury
> - superficial thrombosis.

Remember: [A]
- chronic oedema or venous insufficiency
- pelvic tumours compressing lymphatic or venous drainage
- a ruptured Baker's cyst.

Baker's cyst
- Remember the presence of a Baker's cyst (ruptured or not) does not exclude a DVT. [A]
- Look for: [A]
  + crepitus on flexing the knee
  + a history of arthritis
  + an abnormal ultrasound scan.

In addition, ask about features that might affect your management:
- recurrent venous thromboembolism [A]
- a known clotting disorder [B]
- a history of clotting disorders in first-degree relatives [C]
- use of the oral contraceptive pill [B]
- current or recent pregnancy. [B]

Pregnancy
- A DVT is less likely if only the right leg is affected clinically. [A]
- A DVT is not more likely in any particular trimester. [B]

INVESTIGATIONS

- Blood count. [D]
- Clotting. [D]
- Thrombophilia studies if indicated. [C]

Thrombophilia screen
Patient aged < 41, and a family history of thrombophilia: [C]
- factor V_{Leiden}
- protein C
- protein S
- plasminogen
- antiphospholipid antibiodies.

− D-dimer in low-risk patients. [A]

Note
A negative D-dimer can help rule out a DVT in low-risk cases. [A]

± Ultrasound scan. Base further investigations on the following plan. [A]

DVT probability	Ultrasound result	Further investigation, if required
High	Ultrasound • positive: DVT • negative: venogram	Venogram • positive: DVT • negative: no DVT
Moderate	Ultrasound • positive: DVT • negative: repeat scan in 1 week and withhold anticoagulation [A]	Repeat ultrasound • positive: DVT • negative: no DVT
Low	Ultrasound • positive: venogram • negative: no DVT	Venogram • positive: DVT • negative: no DVT

Ultrasound
- Arrange for compression ultrasound scanning of the common femoral and popliteal veins to the trifurcation. The test is positive if any vein is not fully compressible. [A]
- Ultrasound scans can diagnose recurrent DVT in patients with a recent DVT. [A]

Alternatives are:
± Impedance plethysmography [A] preferably with a D-dimer. [A] Base further investigations on the following plan. [A]

DVT probability	IPG result	Further investigation, if required
High	IPG • positive: DVT • negative: venogram	Venogram • positive: DVT • negative: no DVT
Moderate	IPG • positive: DVT • negative: repeat scan in 1 week and withhold anticoagulation	Repeat ultrasound • positive: DVT • negative: no DVT
Low	IPG • positive: venogram • negative: no DVT	Venogram • positive: DVT • negative: no DVT

Impedance plethysmography
- IPG is less effective than ultrasonography at diagnosing or excluding DVT.
- IPG scans can diagnose recurrent DVT in patients with a recent DVT. [A]

± Venography. [A]

Venography
It is the current reference standard, but:
- some DVTs are missed [C]
- 5% of cases are not technically possible [C]
- pain is a common side-effect [C]
- it may cause DVT. [C]

± MRI [B] from the popliteal veins to the inferior vena cava.

Note
Avoid fibrinogen leg scanning – it cannot safely diagnose or exclude a DVT. [C]

THERAPY

- Give analgesia if necessary.
- Start anticoagulation [A] in all suspected cases [D] using a low-molecular weight heparin. [D]
- Start warfarin [A] as soon as a deep vein thrombosis has been demonstrated. [D]
- Stop the oral contraceptive pill or HRT. [D]
- Ask patients to wear knee-length sized-to-fit elasticated stockings during the day. [A]

Low-molecular weight heparins
- dalteparin 200 units/kg daily
- enoxaparin 1 mg/kg twice daily
- tinzaparin 175 units/kg once daily
- give LMWH [D] for a minimum of 5 days, and continue for 2 days after the INR is within therapeutic range. [D]

See Chapter 19 for more details on LMWH and warfarin dosing.

REVIEW

- Anticoagulation can be completed on an outpatient basis in uncomplicated cases. [A]
- Monitor INR levels daily until warfarin dosing is stable. [D]

- Check the platelet count after 5 days. If it is $< 150 \times 10^9/L$, then repeat the test. If confirmed, treat for heparin-induced thrombocytopenia. [A]
- Continue warfarin:
  - for 6 weeks for transient risk factors, [A] e.g. surgery, trauma
  - for 6 months for permanent risk factors, e.g. cancer, leg paralysis
  - indefinitely
    - for idiopathic cases [A]
    - for recurrent venous thromboembolism. [A]

Avoid outpatient anticoagulation in patients with: [D]
- recurrent venous thromboembolism
- active bleeding
- a clotting disorder
- problems being followed up.

Therapeutic ranges

Indication	Target INR
Venous thromboembolism [C]	2.0 to 3.0
Venous thromboembolism when INR 2.0 to 3.0 [D]	3.0 to 4.5

Outcomes
- Half of patients have a silent PE, [B] though few develop serious problems if anticoagulated. [A]
- A quarter have recurrent venous thromboembolism within 5 years, [A] particularly with cancer or a clotting disorder. [A]
- A quarter develop post-thrombotic leg within 5 years. [A]
- A quarter die within 5 years, [A] particularly with cancer. [A]
- Roughly 1% of patients are diagnosed with a cancer in the next year. [C]

VENOUS THROMBOEMBOLISM PROPHYLAXIS

Note
- Venous thromboembolism reduces DVT, but increases the risk of having an episode of excessive bleeding or requiring a blood tranfusion. [A]
- It reduces fatal PE without clearly increasing death from haemorrhage. [A]

Give venous thromboembolism prophylaxis to all patients who are:
- having major surgery (especially orthopaedic): [A]
- likely to have poor mobility: [A]
  - major trauma [A]
  - leg plaster cast [A]
  - spinal cord injury [A]
  - stroke [A]
  - decompensated heart failure [A]
  - myocardial infarction or unstable angina [A]
- at increased risk for DVT:
  - old patients in hospital [A]
  - active cancer during chemotherapy [A]
  - patients with recurrent venous thromboembolism in hospital [A]
  - pregnant with thrombophilia. [A]

Use:

Low-risk cases
- Thigh-length compression stockings. [A]

Moderate-risk cases
- Thigh-length compression stockings [A] with [A] low-dose heparin [A] 5000 units s.c. every 12 hours.

High-risk cases
- Thigh-length compression stockings [A] with [A] any of:
  - low-molecular weight heparin, [A] e.g. enoxaparin 40 mg daily
  - thigh-length intermittent pneumatic compression [A]
  - warfarin. [A]

Alternatives include:
- hirudin [A]
- anti-platelet drugs. [A]

Continue prophylaxis for as long as the patient is at risk. [A]

Expires July 2003   Guideline: Chris Ball
                      CATs: Chris Ball, Clare Wootton

17
DELIRIUM

SYMPTOMS AND SIGNS

Take a history from the patient, and family members, carers or the patient's primary physician. D

> **Causes of delirium**
> Common causes of delirium include: B
> - infection: pneumonia, chronic lung disease, urinary tract, meningitis
> - heart failure and ischaemic heart disease
> - gastrointestinal disorders
> - cerebrovascular disease
> - drug overdose or withdrawal of antidepressants, anticonvulsants, digoxin, oral hypoglycaemics
> - cancer
> - diabetes mellitus or other metabolic disorders including hypoglycaemia, hypercalcaemia
> - renal failure
> - anaemia.
>
> Remember: D
> - thyroid disorders
> - CNS disorders:
>   - head trauma
>   - post-ictal state
>   - acute glaucoma
> - pain or discomfort:
>   - urinary retention
>   - faecal impaction
>   - post-operative pain.

Use the following to determine if your patient is confused:
± Confusion assessment method: A
1. Is there evidence of an acute change in mental state from the patient's baseline, with fluctuation during that day (i.e. coming and going, increasing and decreasing in severity)?
2. Does the patient have difficulty focusing attention (e.g. being easily distracted, or difficulty keeping track of what is said)?
3. Is the patient's thinking disorganized or incoherent (e.g. rambling, irrelevant conversation, unclear or illogical flow of ideas, unpredictable switching from subject to subject)?
4. Is the patient other than alert (e.g. hyperalert, lethargic, stupor, coma)?

Diagnose delirium if 1 and 2, and either 3 or 4 are present.

± A mini-mental state examination. ^C Calculate your patient's score using the questions in Table 17.1.

Table 17.1   Mini-mental state examination

Maximum score	Question
5	What is the [year] [season] [date] [day] [month]?
5	Where are we [state/country] [county] [town] [hospital] [floor]?
3	Name 3 objects: 1 second to say each. Then ask the patient to name all 3. Give 1 point for each correct answer. Repeat them until he or she learns all 3. Count trials and record.
5	Serial 7's: 1 point for each correct answer. Stop after 5 answers. Alternatively spell 'world' backwards
3	Ask for the 3 objects repeated above. Give 1 point for each correct answer.
2	Hold up a pen and a watch and ask the patient what each is.
1	Repeat the following: 'no ifs, ands or buts'.
3	Follow a 3-stage command: 'take a paper in your right hand, fold it in half, and put it on the floor'.
1	Have the patient read and obey the following statement: 'Close your eyes'.
1	Write a sentence.
1	Copy a design (e.g. 2 interlinked squares).

Total maximum score is 30.
A score ≥ 29 makes dementia or delirium unlikely.
A score ≤ 23 makes dementia or delirium more likely.

± A 10-point clock test. ^C

10-point clock test
- Draw a circle in your patient's medical chart.
- Ask your patient to write the numbers in the face of a clock, and then make the clock say 10 minutes after 11.
- Score one point each for 1, 2, 4, 5, 7, 8, 10, 11, if at least half of its area is in the proper octant of the circle relevant to the number 12.
- Score one point for a short hand pointing to the number 11 and one point for the long hand pointing to the number 2. Award no points for hands if you are unable to tell at a glance which hand is longer.

A score of ≤ 5 makes delirium or dementia more likely; a score of 10 makes delirium or dementia less likely.

Ask about:
- inadequate fluid intake ^A
- a fall in the last 30 days ^A

- dementia [A] or other CNS disorder [C]
- cancer [C]
- medication, and any recent changes: [A]
  - particularly benzodiazepine use (equivalent to > 5 mg diazepam within the last 5 days) [C]
- alcohol intake. [C]

> **Think about other causes of cognitive impairment**
> - dementia:
>   - Alzheimer type
>   - multi-infarct dementia
>   - dementia associated with Parkinson's disease
> - drug withdrawal, especially alcohol
> - depression or psychosis.

Look for:
- ± hypoxia [C]
- evidence of infection [B]
- evidence of neurological problems [B]
- evidence of GI problems – perform a rectal examination [B]
- evidence of acute glaucoma [B]
- dehydration, looking for: [A]
  - + sunken eyes
  - + dry axillae
  - ± dry nose or mouth mucous membranes
  - ± longitudinal furrow on the tongue
- predisposing factors:
  - visual impairment [A]
  - severe illness [A]
  - cognitive impairment [A]
  - urea : creatinine ratio ≥ 0.075 [A]

Predisposing factors for delirium [A]

Number of factors	Risk of delirium
3 or 4	32%
1 or 2	16%
0	3%

- in hospital patients, look for precipitating factors:
  - use of physical restraints [A]
  - malnutrition (weight loss and fall in serum albumin) [A]
  - > 3 medications added on the previous day [A]
  - use of bladder catheterization [A]
  - any iatrogenic event (e.g. transfusion reactions, bleeding due to over-coagulation etc.). [A]

Precipitating factors for delirium [A]	
Number of factors	Risk of delirium
3 or more	36%
1 or 2	20%
0	4%

INVESTIGATIONS

- Blood count. [C]
- Clotting. [D]
- Glucose. [D]
- Urea, electrolytes, creatinine. [A]
- Liver function tests. [D]
- Calcium, phosphate. [D]
- Thyroid function tests. [B]
- Urine dipstick and culture. [D]
- Blood culture. [D]
- ECG. [D]
- Chest X-ray. [D]

Consider:
- vitamin B_{12}, folate levels [B]
- syphilis serology [B]
- arterial blood gases [D]
- CT scan of the head [D]
- lumbar puncture. [D]

THERAPY

- Treat or remove any underlying cause
- Rehydrate patients – mild dehydration can be corrected with a subcutaneous fluid infusion. [A]
- Correct any electrolyte abnormalities. [D]
- Control agitation with haloperidol. [D]
- Consider vitamin supplements, particularly thiamine. [D]

Preventing delirium [B]
- Orientate the patient using:
  - a board with names of the care-team members and the day's schedule
  - communication to re-orientate
  - cognitively stimulating activities

- Maximize sleep using:
  - sleep protocols, such as a night-time drink, relaxation music, back massage
  - noise reduction
- Mobilize patients early by:
  - providing exercise 3 times a day
  - minimizing use of immobilizing equipment
- Maximize vision and hearing by:
  - using visual aids and adaptive equipment with daily reinforcement of use
  - using hearing aids, earwax disimpaction, and special communication techniques
- Recognize early signs of dehydration and volume depletion, and encourage oral fluids.

REVIEW

- Monitor mental status and behaviour. [D]
- Start rehabilitation early. [D]

Outcomes

- Over half of patients are diagnosed with dementia in the next 2 years. [B]
- One in 20 elderly patients admitted to hospital dies before discharge, rising to one in eight at 3 months. [A]
- One in 12 is newly admitted to a nursing home on discharge, rising to one in nine at 3 months. [A]
- One in four suffers a functional decline in the next 3 months. [A]
- Patients who develop delirium are at increased risk of dying, being newly admitted to a nursing home, or having a functional decline within 3 months. [A]

18
DIABETIC KETOACIDOSIS

SYMPTOMS AND SIGNS

Ask about:
- known diabetes mellitus [B]
- previous episodes of diabetic ketoacidosis [B]
- current medication [A] and any recent changes or mistakes [B]
- recent illness [B]
- polyuria, polydipsia and weakness. [D]

Diabetic ketoacidosis
- hyperglycaemia (> 14 mmol/L)
- metabolic acidosis (pH < 7.35 or bicarbonate < 15 mmol/L)
- high anion gap
- ketonaemia.

Hyperglycaemic hyperosmolar nonketosis
- blood glucose higher (often > 33 mmol/L)
- no acidosis
- ketonuria + at the most on urine dipstick
- higher Na (often > 150 mmol/L).

Note
A quarter of cases are patients with new-onset diabetes mellitus. [C]

Look for: [B]
- dehydration
- infection (e.g. lobar pneumonia, urinary tract infection)
- associated disease (e.g. myocardial infarction, pancreatitis).

Think about acidosis in any hyperventilating patient. [D]

Causes of diabetic ketoacidosis
- infection
- treatment error
- new-onset diabetes
- other medical illnesses:
  - pancreatitis
  - myocardial infarction
  - heart failure
  - GI bleed
- drugs or alcohol
- unknown.

INVESTIGATIONS

- Measure glucose rapidly using reagent strips [A] or a capillary glucose. [A]
- Take a urine sample and test for:
  - ketones [C]
  - leukocytes or nitrites – if abnormal send for culture.[D]
- Blood glucose.
- Urea and electrolytes, creatinine. [C]
- Ketones. [A]
- pH [A] and bicarbonate [C] from arterial or venous blood. [C]
- Blood count. [B]
- Cardiac enzymes. [B]
- Amylase. [B]
- Magnesium, phosphate. [D]
- Blood cultures. [D]
- 12-lead ECG and ECG monitoring. [B]
- Chest X-ray. [B]
- Repeat electrolyte and glucose levels [C] frequently [D] until biochemical normality is achieved.

Anion gap (Na + K – HCO$_3$)
Look for:
± an anion gap > 16 mmol/L [C]
± bicarbonate < 15 mmol/L [C]

Pseudohyponatraemia
- High glucose levels can give falsely low sodium levels.
- A corrected sodium level can be calculated using:
  Na + glucose/3

In dehydrated or comatose patients, consider: [D]
- a central line
- inserting a urinary catheter to monitor urine output. [D]

THERAPY

- Resuscitate and get help if needed. [D]
- Give intravenous fluids [A] – initially 0.9% saline. [C] Try: [D]
  - 1 litre over 30 minutes
  - 1 litre over 1 hour
  - 1 litre over 2 hours
  - 1 litre over 4 hours.

- Give an insulin infusion [A] intravenously. [D]

- Give potassium supplementation [A] after insulin therapy has begun.

- Give broad-spectrum antibiotics if there is evidence of infection, e.g. co-amoxiclav 1.2 g every 8 hours.

- For patients with hyperglycaemic hyperosmolar nonketosis, give heparin 5000 units s.c. every 12 hours. [D]

- Monitor electrolytes [C] and capillary glucose [D] initially hourly, then every 2 hours until stable. [D]

Note

If none of the following are present, fluid can be given more slowly if necessary: [D]
- shock
- oliguria during first 4 hours of admission
- renal failure (urea > 21 mmol/L or creatinine > 350 μmol/L)

An insulin infusion regimen [D]

Add 50 units of actrapid (soluble) insulin to 50 ml of 0.9% saline. Infuse using the following sliding scale.

Glucose mmol/L	Infusion rate units/hr
0 to 4	0.5 and 10% or 20% glucose infusion
4 to 8	1
8 to 12	2
12 to 16	3
16 to 20	4
> 20	6 and call doctor

The regimen may need to be adjusted depending on your patient's response.

Potassium supplementation [D]

Serum K mmol/L	Add the following to i.v. fluid bags
> 4.5	nil
3.5 to 4.5	20 mmol per litre
< 3.5	40 mmol per litre

REVIEW

- Monitor vital signs, electrolytes and urine output. [D]

- Continue the insulin infusion until: [A]
  - glucose < 10 mmol/L
  - ketones are cleared (3-hydroxybutyrate < 0.5 mmol/L).
- Once your patient has stabilized [C] and is eating, [D] swap to subcutaneous insulin.
- Give the first subcutaneous dose, then stop the infusion an hour later if your patient remains well.

- Refer your patient to a diabetes team and educate your patient about diabetes. [A]

Note

Watch out for cerebral oedema among patients aged < 30, particularly with serum sodium concentrations that fail to rise during rehydration. [C]

Note

If glucose < 10 mmol/L but ketones are still raised, continue the insulin infusion with 5% or 10% glucose i.v. to maintain glucose 5 to 10 mmol/L. [C]

Outcomes
- Few patients die – death is mainly from infection or ischaemia. [B]
- Half of patients have another episode. [C]

19
DRUGS

AMINOGLYCOSIDES

Avoid aminoglycosides in patients with:
- renal dysfunction (creatinine clearance < 60 ml/min or rising creatinine)
- shock

unless there is no good alternative. [D]

Estimate your patient's creatinine clearance. [D]

Calculate
- **estimated creatinine clearance** (ml/min):

$$\frac{(140 - age) \times weight\ (kg)}{Cr\ (\mu mol/L)}$$

Multiply by 1.2 for men.

- If the patient is obese, use an estimate of the patient's ideal body weight to calculate creatinine clearance.
- Ideal body weight (kg) for males 52 kg + 0.72 kg for every cm above 154 cm in height.
- Ideal body weight (kg) for females 49 kg + 0.64 kg for every cm above 154 cm in height.

In obese patients, calculate a dose-determining weight. [D]

Dose-determining weight
Ideal body weight + (0.4 × (actual body weight − ideal body weight))

Creatinine clearance > 60 ml/min
- Give aminoglycosides once a day [A] (Gentamicin, usually 4.5 mg/kg of dose-determining weight).
- Monitor levels during therapy and adjust dose intervals. Measure a trough level prior to the third dose. [D] If above trough levels increase the dose interval or reduce the dose. [D]
- Monitor creatinine levels during therapy. [D]

Trough levels
Gentamicin < 2 μg/ml

Creatinine clearance ≤ 60 ml/min

- Adjust the dose or the dose interval according to the level of dysfunction and clinical circumstances. [D]
- Monitor levels during therapy and adjust dose intervals. Measure a trough level prior to the second dose. [D] If above trough levels, increase the dose interval or reduce the dose. [D]
- Monitor creatinine levels daily during therapy. [D]

Expires July 2003   Guideline: Catherine Clase, Chris Ball
                        CATs: Catherine Clase, Chris Ball, Clare Wotton

CONTRAST MEDIA

Use low-osmolality contrast media [A] particularly for high-risk patients, i.e.:
- with pre-existing renal impairment. [B]
- with diabetes mellitus [B]
- undergoing angiography. [B]

Give high-risk patients pre- and post-contrast:
- 0.45% saline 1 ml/kg/h for 12 hours [D]
- acetylcysteine 600 mg twice daily. [A]

Avoid the following drugs near the procedure:
- metformin [D]
- frusemide [A]
- mannitol. [D]

Note

The risk of anaphylaxis following contrast is increased with: [B]
- beta-blockers
- asthma.

Expires July 2003 Guideline: Catherine Clase, Chris Ball
CATs: Catherine Clase, Chris Ball, Clare Wotton

HEPARIN

Indications
Use heparin if LMWH is not available or contraindicated. The indications are the same as those for LMWH.

Dosing and monitoring
- Give heparin subcutaneously [A] using a weight-based regimen (see Table 19.1). [C]

Table 19.1   Subcutaneous heparin regimen

aPTT	Adjustment of heparin dose	Time to next aPTT
< 50 s	One step up	After 6 hours
50 to 90 s	Same step	After 6 hours
91 to 120 s	One step down	After 6 hours
> 120 s	Withhold heparin, perform aPTT and proceed as follows:	
	• < 50 s: same step	After 6 hours
	• 50 to 90 s: one step down	After 6 hours
	• 91 to 120 s: 2 steps down	After 6 hours
	• > 120 s: withhold heparin therapy	After 3 hours

Steps 10 000–12 500–15 000–17 500–21 250–25 000–30 000 units twice daily.

- If heparin is given intravenously, use a weight-based regimen (see Table 19.2). [A]

Table 19.2   Intravenous heparin regimen [A]
Add 25 000 units heparin to 50 ml 0.9% saline.

aPTT ratio	Adjustment of heparin dose
Initially	80 units/kg bolus, then 18 units/kg/h
< 1.2	80 units/kg bolus, then increase by 4 units/kg/h
1.2 to 1.5	80 units/kg bolus, then increase by 2 units/kg/h
1.5 to 2.5	No change
2.3 to 3.0	Decrease rate by 2 units/kg/h
> 3.0	Stop infusion for 1 hour, then decrease rate by 3 units/kg/h

- Use aPTT to monitor – check the levels 6 hours after the initial infusion, then daily. [C]
- Aim for an aPTT ratio of 1.5 to 2.5. [D]
- Check the platelet count after 5 days. If it is < 150 × 10^9/L, then repeat the test. If confirmed, treat for heparin-induced thrombocytopenia. [A]

Complications

Major bleeds
- Stop heparin. [A]
- Give protamine sulphate: maximum dose 50 mg by slow i.v. infusion. [D]

Minor bleeds
- Consider stopping heparin. [D]

Heparin-induced thrombocytopenia
- Stop heparin. [A]
- Use an alternative, such as danaparoid. [D]

Other complications
- subcutaneous haematoma [D]
- osteopenia in prolonged administration. [D]

Expires July 2003   Guideline: Chris Ball
CATs: Chris Ball, Clare Wotton
With thanks to David Keeling, John Reynolds, David Sackett, Sharon Straus, and Alan Townsend for the use of their anticoagulation guide.

LOW-MOLECULAR WEIGHT HEPARIN

Indications

Use low-molecular weight heparin rather than heparin for the following conditions:

- unstable angina [A]
- deep vein thrombosis [A]
- pulmonary embolism [D]
- cardioversion for atrial fibrillation. [D]

> **Note**
> - LMWH give a more predictable dose-response than heparin, so rarely require monitoring. [D]
> - LMWH are given subcutaneously.
> - LMWH are probably safe in pregnant women. [C]

Dosing and monitoring

- Use any low-molecular weight heparin – no clinically significant differences between current drugs have been noted. [D]
- Dose according to the patient's weight and give it subcutaneously. [A]
- Monitoring is not required. [D]
- Check the platelet count after 5 days. If it is $< 150 \times 10^9/L$, then repeat the test. If confirmed, treat for heparin-induced thrombocytopenia. [A]

> **Dosing regimens**
> - dalteparin 200 units/kg daily
> - enoxaparin 1 mg/kg twice daily
> - tinzaparin 175 units/kg once daily.

Complications

Major bleeds
- Stop LMWH. [A]
- Give protamine sulphate: maximum dose 50 mg by slow i.v. infusion. [D]

> **Note**
> - 1 mg protamine inhibits 100 IU dalteparin.
> - Fresh-frozen plasma does not reverse the anticoagulant effect of LMWH.

Minor bleeds
- Consider stopping LMWH. [D]

Heparin-induced thrombocytopenia
- Stop LMWH. [A]
- Use an alternative, such as danaparoid. [D]

Other complications
- subcutaneous haematoma [D]
- osteopenia in prolonged administration. [D]

Expires July 2003 Guideline: Chris Ball
CATs: Chris Ball, Clare Wotton
With thanks to David Keeling, John Reynolds, David Sackett, Sharon Straus, and Alan Townsend for the use of their anticoagulation guide.

WARFARIN

Indications

Give warfarin for the following conditions:
- venous thromboembolism [A]
- atrial fibrillation [A]
- heart valves [A]
- ventricular aneurysm [A]
- anti-phospholipid syndrome. [C]

Therapeutic ranges	
Indication	**Target INR**
Venous thromboembolism [C]	2.0 to 3.0
Venous thromboembolism when INR 2.0 to 3.0 [D]	3.0 to 4.5
Atrial fibrillation [B]	2.0 to 3.0
Biological heart valves [A]	2.0 to 3.0
Mechanical heart valves [B]	3.0 to 4.5

Determine your patient's risk of bleeding on warfarin, before deciding if it is worthwhile. [D] See Table 7.2.

If warfarin is contraindicated consider:
- a vena caval filter for deep vein thrombosis. [D]
- long-term subcutaneous heparin or LMWH. [D]

Dosing and monitoring

- Start warfarin as soon as possible [A] and monitor its effect using INR. [A]
  - In patients with venous thromboembolism, give LMWH or heparin while awaiting satisfactory oral anticoagulation. [A]
  - Give heparin [D] and LMWH [D] for a minimum of 5 days, and continue for 2 days after the INR is within therapeutic range. [D]
- Use a set dosing regimen (preferably by computer [A]) and seek expert advice when indicated. [A] See Table 19.3 for a typical dosing regimen.

Follow-up

- Patients should have their INR levels checked regularly. [A]
- Advise patients:
  - About the risk of bleeding, but indicate that serious bleeds are rare. [B]
  - Most patients on warfarin feel as healthy as patients who are not. [A]
  - Many drugs and foods (including alcohol) interact, and patients should check that any new medication they take is safe. [B]
  - Warfarin can cause fetal abnormalities [A] – women planning to get pregnant should swap to heparin. [D]

Note

Anticoagulation is potentiated by: [B]
- antibiotics and antifungals:
  - co-trimoxazole
  - erythromycin
  - fluconazole
  - isoniazid
  - metronidazole
- cardiac drugs:
  - amiodarone
  - clofibrate
  - propafenone
  - propranolol
  - statins
- analgesics:
  - paracetamol
  - piroxicam
- alcohol
- cimetidine and omeprazole.

Anticoagulation is inhibited by: [B]
- antibiotics and antifungals:
  - griseofulvin
  - rifampicin
  - nafcillin
- CNS drugs:
  - barbiturates
  - carbamazepine
  - chlordiazepoxide
- cholestyramine
- sucralfate
- foods and feeds high in vitamin K.

Note

Monitor patients more closely:
- on 2.5 g or more of paracetamol per week [B]
- recently started on warfarin-potentiating medication [B]
- taking more warfarin than prescribed [B]
- with advanced cancer [B]
- with reduced oral intake in the last week [B]
- with acute diarrhoea in the last week. [B]

Table 19.3 Warfarin dosing regimen to achieve INR 2.0 to 3.0 [B]

- Give warfarin at 5 to 6 p.m. and measure the INR at 9 a.m. the next day.
- Monitor INR daily until in range and stable.

Day	INR	≤ 50 years
1	< 1.4	10
2	< 1.6	10
	≥ 1.6	0.5
3	< 1.8	10
	1.8 to 2.5	4.0 to 5.0
	2.6 to 3.0	2.5 to 3.5
	3.1 to 3.5	1.0 to 2.0
	3.6 to 4.0	0.5
	> 4.0	0
4	< 1.6	10.0 to 15.0
	1.6 to 1.9	6.0 to 8.0
	2.0 to 2.6	4.5 to 5.5
	2.7 to 3.5	3.5 to 4.0
	3.6 to 4.0	3
	4.1 to 4.5	
		1.0 to 2.0
	> 4.5	

Decrease the dose by 33% if the patient has one or more of the following risk factors:
- severe congestive heart failure (ejection fraction < 30% and/or biventricular failure)
- severe chronic obstructive airways disease (oxygen or steroid use or dyspnoea at rest)
- concurrent amiodarone use.

Complications

Life-threatening bleed

- Give 5 mg vitamin K by slow i.v. infusion. [A]
- Give factor concentrate or FFP. [C]
- Stop warfarin. [C]

Major bleed

- Stop warfarin for 1 or more days. [C]
- Consider giving 0.5 to 2.0 mg vitamin K i.v. [C]

INR > 5.0 without haemorrhage

- Continue warfarin and give 2 mg of vitamin K orally. [A]

Dose for age (mg)		
51 to 65 years	**66 to 80 years**	**> 80 years**
9	7.5	6
9	7.5	6
0.5	0.5	0.5
9	7.5	6
3.5 to 4.5	3.0 to 4.0	2.5 to 3.0
2.5 to 3.5	2.0 to 2.5	1.5 to 2.0
1.0 to 2.0	0.5 to 1.5	0.5 to 1.5
0.5	0.5	0
0	0	0
9.0 to 13.0	7.5 to 11.0	6.0 to 9.0
5.5 to 7.0	4.5 to 6.0	3.5 to 5.0
4.0 to 5.0	3.5 to 4.5	2.5 to 3.5
3.0 to 3.5	2.5 to 3.0	2.0 to 2.5
2.5	2	1.5
	Omit next day's dose then	
1.0 to 2.0	1.0 to 2.0	1.0 to 2.0
	zdose	

Unexpected bleeding at therapeutic levels of INR

- Investigate for underlying malignancy – particularly GI and GU neoplasms. [B]

Rare complications
- warfarin-induced skin necrosis. [D]

Expires July 2003 Guideline: Chris Ball
CATs: Chris Ball, Clare Wotton
With thanks to David Keeling, John Reynolds, David Sackett, Sharon Straus, and Alan Townsend for the use of their anticoagulation guide.

20
GIANT CELL ARTERITIS

SYMPTOMS AND SIGNS

Ask about:
- − recent onset headache [B]
- + jaw claudication [B]
- + anorexia [C]
- ■ tongue claudication [C]
- ■ visual disturbances [D]
- ■ a history of polymyalgia rheumatica. [D]

> **Note**
> - Tongue claudication makes giant cell arteritis less likely. [C]
> - If there is no recent-onset headache, jaw claudication or abnormal temporal artery, then giant cell arteritis is unlikely. [B]

> **Think about giant cell arteritis in patients aged > 50 presenting with any of:** [D]
> - headache
> - malaise
> - jaw pains
> - scalp tenderness
> - visual changes.

Look for:
- ± an abnormal temporal artery (hot, red, tender) [A]
- ■ complications, e.g. vision loss, stroke, neuropathy [D]
- ■ other causes of headache.

> **Think about other causes**
> - infection: meningitis
> - stroke or intracranial haemorrhage
> - connective tissue disease
> - migraine or cluster headache
> - non-specific headache.

INVESTIGATIONS

- + Blood count. [C]
- ± ESR or plasma viscosity. [A]

Note
- An ESR > 60 mm/h or plasma viscosity > 1.8 helps diagnose giant cell arteritis. [A]
- Around 20% of patients have a normal ESR when first seen. [A]

■ U&E, creatinine. [D]
■ ECG. [D]
± Arrange for a bilateral [C] temporal artery biopsy [A] in areas of pain or inflammation. [C]

Note
Patients with negative biopsies who meet all the following criteria should be diagnosed with giant cell arteritis: [D]
1. aged > 55
2. a positive response to steroids within 48 hours
3. a history lasting > 2 weeks
4. at least 3 of the following:
   - proximal and symmetrical girdle or upper arm muscle pain, stiffness or tenderness
   - jaw claudication
   - clinically abnormal temporal artery (tender, thickened, red)
   - systemic symptoms or signs (malaise, anorexia, weight loss, anaemia, pyrexia)
   - recent-onset headache
   - visual disturbance (loss, dip, blurring).

THERAPY

Give corticosteroids [A] immediately in all suspected cases. [D] Start with 40 mg prednisolone [D] daily [A] with:
- vitamin D and calcium supplements [A]
- oral methotrexate 10 mg weekly. [A]

Steroids
- Warn your patient about the possible need for long-term steroid therapy, and that side-effects are common with long-term use.
- Mention: [C]
  - weight gain
  - osteoporosis
  - Cushing's syndrome
  - hypertension
  - diabetes mellitus
  - dyspepsia.

Consider starting:
- antacid medication if patients complain of dyspepsia [A]
- bisphosphonates. [A]

REVIEW

- Warn patients about the possibility of relapse. [A]
- Monitor ESR, but discharge patients only when symptoms have improved. [D]

Outcomes
- 60–80% of patients relapse within 2 years [B] – half are triggered by attempting to reduce the steroid dose. [C]
- ESR or CRP alone do not usefully predict which patients relapse or develop complications, so adjust the dose based on your patient's symptoms. [D]
- Vision loss is permanent. [C]
- Patients are at risk of strokes and other vessel disease. [C]

21
CONGESTIVE HEART FAILURE

SYMPTOMS AND SIGNS

Ask about:
+ a previous myocardial infarction [B]
+ previous episodes of congestive heart failure [A]
+ orthopnoea [B]
− dyspnoea on exertion [B]
■ current medication and alcohol use. [D]

> **Think about other causes of dypsnoea**
> - asthma
> - COPD
> - arrhythmia
> - infection
> - interstitial lung disease
> - anaemia
> - pulmonary embolism.

Look for:
+ tachycardia [B]
+ dyspnoea [B]
+ hypotension or hypertension [B]
+ oedema. [B]
+ an elevated jugular venous pressure [B]
+ a displaced apical pulse [A]
+ an abnormal abdominojugular reflex. [B]

> **Abdominojugular reflex**
> Ask the patient to relax and breathe through an open mouth. Place the palm of your hand on the mid-abdomen and push at a pressure of 20 to 35 mmHg for 15 to 30 seconds:
> - positive if sustained increase in JVP ≥ 4cm
> - negative if sustained increase ≤ 3cm, or transient increase ≥ 4cm.
> Repeat the test if there is pain, or if the patient holds his breath or bears down.

Listen for:
+ added heart sounds [B] or a gallop rhythm [B]
+ murmurs [B]
+ crackles on chest examination. [B]

Causes of heart failure D
- fluid overload
- pulmonary embolism
- pump failure:
  - myocardial infarction
  - valvular heart disease
  - constrictive pericarditis
  - myocarditis
- arrhythmias
- drugs and others
  - NSAIDs
  - beta-blockers
  - alcohol
  - thiamine deficiency
- increased demands:
  - pregnancy
  - fever
  - hyperthyroidism
  - anaemia
  - accelerated hypertension.

INVESTIGATIONS

- Blood count. D
- U&E, creatinine. A
- Glucose. B
- Cardiac enzymes. D
- Thyroid function tests. D
- Arterial blood gas if dyspnoeic. D
- ECG. B
- Chest X-ray. B

ECG changes
Look for:
+ anterior Q waves B
+ left bundle-branch block. B

Chest X-ray changes
Look for:
+ cardiomegaly B
+ upper lobe bloodflow diversion B
+ even distribution of oedema B
− normal or wide vascular pedicle width. B

Consider:
- inserting a urinary catheter to monitor urine output [D]
- an echocardiogram [D]
- daily weights. [D]

THERAPY

- Sit your patient upright. [D]
- Oxygen. [A]
- Salbutamol 5 mg [D] and ipratropium 500 μg [B] nebulizers if wheezy.
- Morphine in small doses (2.5 mg i.v.) if very dyspnoeic. [A]
- Frusemide 40 mg to 80 mg [A] intravenously, [D] and continued once or twice daily. [D] Ask patients to remain in bed afterwards. [B] For large doses, consider using an infusion. [D]

For pulmonary oedema:
- Add high-dose isosorbide dinitrate. [A]

Isosorbide dinitrate [A]
- Give a 3 mg bolus of isosorbide dinitrate i.v. every 3 minutes until the oxygen saturation is 96% or the mean arterial blood pressure falls by ≥ 30% or below 90 mmHg.

Consider:
- continuous positive airway pressure (CPAP) for respiratory failure [A]
- inotropic support if there is hypotension. [D] Try dobutamine. [D]

Dobutamine
- Add 250 mg dobutamine to 50 ml 0.9% saline.
- Infuse via a central line at 2 to 10 μg/kg/min (0.024 to 0.12 ml/kg/h).
- Monitor:
  - blood pressure, pulse
  - ECG for ischaemia
  - urine output.

REVIEW

- Start an ACE inhibitor [A] or losartan [A] 50 mg daily.
- Monitor renal function carefully. [D]
- Swap patients to oral medication as symptoms improve. [D]
- Add a thiazide (bendrofluazide 2.5 mg daily or metolazone 1 mg daily) in resistant cases. [C]

ACE inhibitors
- Monitor the blood pressure for the first dose. [D]
- Increase the dose if patients tolerate it. [A]
- Typical doses:
  - Enalapril 2.5 to 5 mg daily initially, increasing to 10 to 20 mg daily.
  - Perindopril 1 mg daily initially, increasing to 4 to 8 mg daily.
  - Ramipril 1.25 mg daily initially, increasing to 5 mg daily. [A]

Consider giving patients with severe left ventricular dysfunction:
- digoxin (even with a normal sinus rhythm) [A]

Digoxin
- Load patients with 500 to 1000 μg in divided doses.
- Give 62.5 to 250 μg daily, based on age, renal function and other medication.
- Measure digoxin levels after 5 days. [D] Take the blood test 6 to 10 hours after the last dose.
- Therapeutic range 0.8 to 2.0 ng/ml.

- spironolactone [A] 25 to 50 mg orally daily
- amiodarone [A]

Amiodarone
Loading dose:
- intravenous: preferably via a central line
  - Give 300 mg (5 mg/kg) in 250 ml 5.0% glucose over 1 hour, followed by 900 mg over 24 hours.

- oral:
  - Give 200 mg every 8 hours for 1 week, then 200 mg every 12 hours for 1 week, then start maintenance therapy.

Maintenance dose:
- Patients should be given a total loading dose of 4200 mg before starting on maintenance therapy. [D]
- Give 100 to 200 mg daily.

- a beta-blocker [A] once stable, [D] e.g. metoprolol 12.5 mg twice daily increasing to 50 mg three times a day if tolerated, or carvedilol 6.25 mg twice daily increasing to 25 mg twice daily if tolerated.
- Arrange a visit by a nurse and a pharmacist to assess the need for further intervention after discharge. [A]

Consider:
- Amlodipine 5 mg daily for dilated cardiomyopathy. [A]

Outcomes

- Readmission is common. [B]
- One in seven dies within a year, [B] often suddenly. [A] The risk is increased with worsening heart failure. [A]
- One in seven with acute pulmonary oedema dies in hospital. [A]

Expires July 2003 Guideline: Chris Ball
CATs: Ati Yates, Chris Ball, Clare Wotton

22
HYPERCALCAEMIA

SYMPTOMS AND SIGNS

Many patients are asymptomatic. Clinical features can be non-specific.

Ask about:
- known malignancy
- current medication, which might:
  - exacerbate hypercalcaemia (thiazides, vitamin D)
  - be more toxic (digoxin). D

Look for: C
- dehydration
- polyuria
- gastrointestinal symptoms (nausea, vomiting, constipation)
- confusion and psychiatric symptoms
- bony pain D
- evidence of urinary calculi. D

Look for a cause A e.g. evidence of malignancy.

> **Common causes include:** C
> - primary hyperparathyroidism
> - malignancy
> - renal failure.
>
> **Rarer causes include:**
> - sarcoidosis
> - thyrotoxicosis
> - excessive vitamin D therapy.

INVESTIGATIONS

- Calcium. A
- Albumin. A
- Alkaline phosphatase. D
- Urea, electrolytes. C
- Phosphate. C
- Magnesium. C
- Thyroid function tests. C
- ± Parathyroid hormone. C
- + PTH-related protein. C
- ECG. D
- Chest X-ray. D

> **Corrected calcium**
> Adjust calcium for the albumin level:
> - corrected calcium (mmol/L) = uncorrected calcium (mmol/L) + (0.02 × (40 − albumin)). [A]

Consider:
- central venous pressure monitoring
- a urethral catheter.

THERAPY

- Resuscitate with i.v. fluids, [A] e.g. 0.9% saline. [D]
- Give frusemide 40–80 mg i.v. [C]

Malignancy

- If normocalcaemia has not been achieved or is unlikely to be achieved after 24 hours, [D] give pamidronate [A] 90 mg i.v. over 1 hour. [A] An alternative is gallium nitrate (200 mg/m² i.v. per day for 5 days). [A]
- Give steroids to patients with steroid-responsive malignancy (e.g. breast cancer, myeloma, renal cell carcinoma). [D]
- Consider arranging dialysis for patients with severe renal insufficiency. [D]

Primary hyperparathyroidism

- Treat asymptomatic and mild cases conservatively. [A]
- Consider hormone replacement therapy in post-menopausal women. [C]
- Refer symptomatic cases for parathyroidectomy. [A]

> **Parathyroidectomy**
> - One in 10 develops hypothyroidism. [A]
> - One in 20 has a permanently hoarse voice. [A]
> - Surgery fails to lower calcium levels in one in 50. [A]

REVIEW

- Monitor electrolytes, calcium and phosphate. [A]

Malignancy

- Give pamidronate infusions (60–90 mg) regularly (every 2 to 4 weeks). [A]
- Arrange radiotherapy for localized bone pain. [A]

> **Outcomes**
> - Recurrent hypercalcaemia is common. [A]
> - Survival is poor in patients with bony metastases. [A]

23
HYPERKALAEMIA

SYMPTOMS AND SIGNS

Patients can present with:
- no specific clinical features [D]
- non-specific weakness and paraesthesias [D]
- sudden cardiac arrest. [D]

Ask about: [B]
- renal failure and look at recent U&E tests
- heart failure
- current medication: specifically ACE inhibitors, infusions, diuretics, NSAIDs.

> **Causes of hyperkalaemia** [C]
> - haemolysis:
>   - poor venepuncture
>   - blood dyscrasias
> - impaired renal function
> - drug treatment:
>   - i.v. infusion
>   - ACE inhibitor
>   - K-sparing drugs
>   - NSAIDs
> - redistribution of potassium:
>   - acidosis
>   - mineralocorticoid deficiency.

INVESTIGATIONS

- Recheck potassium if haemolysis is possible [C] (but get an ECG anyway)
- 12-lead ECG [B] and consider continuous ECG monitoring. [D]

> **ECG changes**
> Look for: [B]
> - peaked T waves, small P waves
> - or worse yet
>   - absent P waves
>   - wide QRS
>   - blurring of ST into T.
>
> The signs are subtle and easy to miss.

If no obvious cause can be found, perform the following investigations: [D]
- blood count
- glucose
- arterial blood gas
- cortisol level
- monitor urine output.

THERAPY

K 6.0–6.5 mmol/L [D] and no ECG changes
- Monitor the patient and correct the cause.

All other cases [D]
- Give 10 ml of 10% calcium gluconate if urgent correction is required (e.g. significant ECG changes). [D]
- Give salbutamol 5 mg by nebulizer [A] with [B] 20 ml of 50% glucose intravenously [B] and short-acting insulin 10 units i.v. over 10 minutes. [B]
- Correct the cause. [D]

REVIEW

- Monitor the serum potassium, and repeat therapy if necessary. [D]
- Refer for dialysis if hyperkalaemia persists or renal function is poor. [A]
- If this is unavailable within a few hours: give calcium resonium. [A]

Watch out for:
- arrhythmias. [D]

Outcomes
- One in seven dies in hospital. [C]

24
HYPERTENSIVE CRISIS

SYMPTOMS AND SIGNS

Repeat the blood pressure to confirm. [D]

> **Hypertensive crisis**
> - diastolic blood pressure ≥ 120 mmHg.
>
> **Hypertensive emergency**
> - as above *plus* evidence of end-organ damage.

Ask patients with known hypertension:
- if they have a GP [B]
- if they take their antihypertensive medication. [B]

> **Common causes include:** [C]
> - essential hypertension
> - renovascular disease
> - diabetic nephropathy
> - neurogenic disease
> - phaechromocytoma
> - primary hyperaldosteronism
> - drugs (cocaine, amphetamine, LSD, phencyclidine) [D]
> - collagen-vascular disease [D]
> - pre-eclampsia [D]
> - spinal cord syndromes. [D]

Ask about:
± headaches, palpitations or sweating attacks. [C]

> **Note**
> The triad of headaches, palpitations and sweating attacks helps diagnose phaechromocytoma. If none is present, a phaechromocytoma is much less likely. [C]

Look for evidence of end-organ damage:
- headache
- psychomotor agitation
- epistaxis
- chest pain
- dyspnoea
- arrhythmias.

Concentrate on excluding the following conditions:
- neurological: [D]
    - cerebral infarction or haemorrhage
    - hypertensive encephalopathy
- cardiovascular:
    - acute pulmonary oedema
    - acute MI or unstable angina
    - aortic dissection
    - coarctation of the aorta
    - renovascular hypertension
- eclampsia.

Perform fundoscopy. [C]

Hypertensive retinal changes [C]	
Grade	**Retinal changes**
I	Minimal changes, no haemorrhages
II	Sclerosis of arterioles ± haemorrhages
III	Exudates ± haemorrhages
IV	Papilloedema

Listen for an abdominal bruit. [A]

Note
Abdominal bruits make renovascular disease more likely. [A]

INVESTIGATIONS

- Urinalysis and urgent microscopy. [B] Look for or request examination for:
    - ± dysmorphic red blood cells [B] (if glomerular disease suspected)
    - − pigmented granular (or haem-granular) casts [B] (if intestinal disease suspected).

Note
Absence of blood or protein on urine dipstick makes glomerular disease less likely. [B]

- Blood count (including MCV and blood film). [D]
- U&E, creatinine. [C]
- Glucose. [C]
- ECG. [C]
- Chest X-ray. [D]

> **Note**
> Potassium < 4.0 mmol/L helps diagnose primary hyperaldosteronism. ᶜ
> Levels greater than this make it less likely, though it may occur with normal
> levels. ᶜ

Consider:
- a head CT if a stroke is suspected
± renin and aldosterone levels ᶜ if primary hyperaldosteronism is suspected
+ plasma catecholamines and a 24-hour urine catecholamine collection ᶜ if a
  phaechromocytoma is suspected
- a renal ultrasound if renovascular disease is suspected. ᴰ

THERAPY

- Repeat blood pressure readings frequently. ᴰ
- Try any of:
  - nifedipine MR 5 mg orally chewed then swallowedᴰ
  - nicardipine 30 mg orally ᴬ
  - enalapril 0.625 mg orally ᶜ or captopril 25 mg sublingually ᴬ
  - labetalol orally ᴰ 100 mg
  - clonidine orally ᴬ 50 μg.

Start patients on regular antihypertensive medication. ᴬ

> **Note**
> - If there is evidence of end-organ damage, aim to reduce the blood
>   pressure immediately. Otherwise aim for a gradual reduction over
>   24 hours. ᴰ
> - Avoid reducing the blood pressure too rapidly. Aim for a reduction to a
>   diastolic < 120 mmHg or a fall > 20 mmHg. ᴰ
> - The indications for parenteral therapy (usually with short-acting and
>   titratable agents) are unclear. Seek help if you think this is indicated. ᴰ

REVIEW

> **Outcomes**
> - A third are dead within 3 years mainly from renal failure or a stroke. ᴮ
> - Few patients end up on dialysis, ᴮ unless they have glomerulonephritis. ᴬ

Expires July 2003 Guideline: Chris Ball, Nick Shenker
                      CATs: Chris Ball, Clare Wotton, Nick Shenker

25
HYPOGLYCAEMIA

SYMPTOMS AND SIGNS

Ask about:
+ diabetes mellitus, [A] particularly:
  + about the current insulin regimen (whether intensive or not) [A]
  + is the disease long-standing [B]
  + about poor glycaemic control [A]
+ any previous episodes of hypoglycaemia [B]
+ current medication, particularly oral hypoglycaemics, [B] beta-blockers, [B] or ACE inhibitors [B]
+ any cardiac problems. [B]

Causes of hypoglycaemia include:
- diabetes mellitus, usually with:
  - a missed meal
  - an insulin overdose
  - alcohol
  - exercise
- alcohol
- attempted suicide
- drugs (beta-blockers, oral hypoglycaemics)
- renal failure.

Look for symptoms of hypoglycaemia: [C]
+ sweating
+ altered consciousness or confusion
+ aggression
■ tachycardia. [D]

Think about hypoglycaemia in patients with:
- a reduced level of consciousness [C]
- hemiparesis [C]
- seizures [C]
- bizarre or aggressive behaviour. [D]

Note
Absence of symptoms does not exclude hypoglycaemia. [C]

INVESTIGATIONS

- Measure glucose rapidly using reagent strips [A] or a capillary glucose. [A]
- Send a blood glucose. [D]
- If you believe hypoglycaemia is present, try a test dose of 50% glucose i.v. (20 to 50 ml). [A]

> **Note**
> Patients with diabetes may develop hypoglycaemic symptoms at 'normoglycaemic' levels. [C]

THERAPY

- If your patient is semi-conscious, [D] give 50% glucose i.v. (20 to 50 ml), [A] or glucagon 0.5 to 1 unit i.m. or i.v. [C]
- If conscious, [D] give a sugary drink. [C]
- Follow any urgent measure with long-acting carbohydrate. [D]

> **Note**
> If there is no response to glucagon, give i.v. glucose. [A]

REVIEW

- Refer to a diabetes team and educate your patient about diabetes. [A]
- Most patients can be safely discharged home on recovery. [D] However, admit a patient with a severe episode (particularly due to oral hypoglycaemics) for blood glucose monitoring. [D]

> **Outcomes**
> - Headache is common on recovery. [B]
> - Recurrence is common, [B] particularly with an intensive insulin regimen, previous episodes of hypoglyacaemia or a low HbA_{1c}. [B]
> - Multiple episodes of hypoglycaemia can lead to brain damage. [C]

26
HYPONATRAEMIA

SYMPTOMS AND SIGNS

Ask about:
- recent illness:
  - diarrhoea and vomiting [C]
  - sweating [C]
- fluid intake [D]
- current medical problems, including:
  - heart failure [C]
  - renal disease [C]
  - liver failure and ascites [C]
  - diabetes mellitus [C]
  - any psychiatric problems [C]
- current medication (particularly diuretics, NSAIDs, antibiotics). [C]

Common causes of hyponatraemia

Chronic causes:
- diuretics
- SIADH
- oedema
- chronic renal failure
- Addison's disease.

Acute causes:
- parenteral fluids and SIADH
- psychogenic polydipsia
- Addison's disease.

Look for:
- evidence of dehydration. [C] Look for: [A]
  - **+** sunken eyes
  - **+** dry axillae
  - **±** dry nose or mouth mucous membranes
  - **±** longitudinal furrows on the tongue
- evidence of oedema. Look for:
  - **+** an elevated jugular venous pressure [B]
  - **+** a displaced apical pulse [A]
  - **+** an abnormal abdominojugular reflex. [B]

> **Note**
> Patients may have nausea, cramps, confusion or seizures. However, unless the serum sodium is falling rapidly, levels in the range 125 to 135 mmol/L are usually asymptomatic. [D]

> **Note**
> The following features are not very helpful at diagnosing dehydration: [B]
> • postural changes in pulse or blood pressure.
> • neurological signs or symptoms (including confusion or slurred speech).

Causes of hyponatraemia
Refer to Table 26.1.

Table 26.1   Causes of hyponatraemia

Dehydration present	No dehydration or oedema present	Oedema present
Renal losses	**Artefact**	
• diuretics	• sample taken from i.v. arm	• congestive heart failure
• adrenal insufficiency	• pseudohyponatraemia	• nephrotic syndrome
• osmotic diuresis (glucose, urea, mannitol)	• hyperglycaemia	• cirrhosis
• renal tubular acidosis	• hypertriglyceridaemia	• renal failure
	• hyperproteinaemia	
Fluid losses	**Acute onset**	
• vomiting, diarrhoea	• excessive i.v. intake post-operatively	
• sweating	• psychogenic polydipsia	
	Chronic onset	
	• syndrome of inappropriate ADH secretion (see below)	
	• hypothyroidism	
	• glucocorticoid deficiency	
	• pain, emotion or drugs	

Syndrome of inappropriate ADH secretion
Diagnose when all the following are present:
■ a low serum sodium
■ a concentrated urine and dilute plasma (urine osmolality > 100 mOsm/kg; plasma osmolality < 270 mOsm/kg)

- a normal circulating volume (no postural hypotension, normal CVP, no pre-renal failure)
- normal renal, adrenal and thyroid function.

Causes include:
- malignancy: small cell bronchus, bladder, pancreas, brain
- infections: pneumonia, CNS, tuberculosis
- brain injury: stroke, tumour, haemorrhage, Guillain–Barré syndrome
- drugs: commonly diuretics, carbamazepine, psychotropics, chlorpropamide.

INVESTIGATIONS

- U&E, creatinine. [A]
- Glucose. [D]
- Serum osmolality.[A]

If indicated: [D]
- Cortisol.
- Thyroid function tests.
- Chest X-ray.

Consider sending a urine sample for biochemistry:
- Urine sodium. [C]
- Urine chloride. [C]
- Urine creatinine. [D]
- Urine osmolality. [C]

Urine biochemistry
Pre-renal failure is more likely with: [C]
- urine sodium < 10 mmol/L
- urine chloride < 10 mmol/L
- urine osmolality > 500 mOsm/kg.

These indices are only valid if patients are not on diuretics and had previously normal renal function.

THERAPY

- Treat the underlying cause. [A] Ask for specialist advice if hyponatraemia fails to correct or recurs. [D]

Note
Aim to correct sodium levels at 0.5 mmol/L per hour with a maximum rise of 12 mmol/L in 24 hours. [D]

Dehydration
- Give 0.9% saline slowly. [C]

Oedema
- Give frusemide 40 mg i.v. [B] and monitor fluid balance carefully.

No dehydration or oedema
- Restrict water intake to 1.5 litres/day, [D] then 1 litre/day if no response. [D]
- Consider demeclocycline 300 mg 8-hourly if no response. [D]

REVIEW

- Monitor electrolytes regularly. [D]
- Monitor fluid balance. [D]

Outcomes
- One in 12 patients with severe hyponatraemia (Na < 110 mmol/l) dies. [C]
- Half of patients with acute severe hyponatraemia (onset < 12 hours) die. [C]
- One in nine develops neurological complications, particularly with severe hyponatraemia or rapid correction. [C]

Expires July 2003 Guideline: Tim Ringrose, Chris Ball
CATs: Tim Ringrose, Chris Ball, Clare Wotton

27
INFECTIVE ENDOCARDITIS

SYMPTOMS AND SIGNS

Ask about:
- valvular heart disease [B] including mitral valve prolapse [B] in particular:
  - which valves are affected [B]
  - the severity of disease [B]
  - any recent valvular surgery (in the last 2 months) [A]
  - any prosthetic valves [B]
- previous rheumatic fever [B]
- previous episodes of endocarditis [B]
- intravenous drug use [B]
- any infectious episode in the last 3 months, [B] particularly superficial wound infections [A] or skin wounds. [B]

> **Note**
> Think about infective endocarditis in patients with:
> - new prosthetic valves [A]
> - bacteraemia. [C]
>
> It is uncommon, but easy to miss! [C]

Look for: [C]
- fever
- rigors
- a new or changed heart murmur
- complications:
  - neurological involvement (headache, mental state changes)
  - emboli: strokes, petechiae (including palettal haemorrhages, Janeway lesions, conjunctival haemorrhages including Roth spots, mycotic aneurysms)
  - evidence of heart failure
  - hepatomegaly
  - splenomegaly.

> **Note**
> - Recent dental, surgical or medical procedures do not clearly increase the risk of developing infective endocarditis. [B]
> - Splinter haemorrhages are unhelpful in diagnosing infective endocarditis. [C]

INVESTIGATIONS

- Blood count [C] with differential. [C]
- U&E, creatinine. [C]
- CRP. [C]
- Liver function tests. [C]
- Blood cultures: [A] at least 3 sets [C] and preferably more, [D] drawn at least 1 hour apart. [D] Save blood for serological investigation in case of 'culture negative' endocarditis. [C]

Blood cultures
Remember to change the needle before inoculating culture bottles. [B]

- Urine dipstick for haematuria. [C]
- ECG. [B]

ECG changes
Look for: [B]
- AV blocks
- bundle branch or fascicular blocks.

These make perivalvular abscesses more likely.

- Chest X-ray. [C]
- Echocardiography (preferably transoesophageal) looking for vegetations. [B]

Use the Duke criteria to establish the diagnosis (see below). [B]

Duke criteria for infective endocarditis [B]

Definite
Any of:
- Pathological criteria:
  - micro-organism: demonstrated by culture of histology in a vegetation, or in a vegetation that has embolized or in an intracardiac abscess, or
  - pathological lesions: vegetation or intracardiac abscess present confirmed by histology showing active endocarditis.
- Clinical criteria: any of (see below for definitions)
  - two major criteria
  - one major and three minor criteria
  - five minor criteria.

Possible
- Findings consistent with infective endocarditis that fall short of 'definite' but not 'rejected'.

Rejected

Any of:

- Firm alternative diagnosis explaining evidence of infective endocarditis syndrome.
- Resolution of infective endocarditis syndrome with antibiotic treatment for < 4 days.
- No pathological evidence of infective endocarditis at surgery or autopsy with antibiotic therapy for < 4 days.

Clinical criteria: major criteria

1. Positive blood culture for infective endocarditis:
   - typical micro-organisms for infective endocarditis from two separate blood cultures:
     - viridans streptococci, *Streptococcus bovis*, HACEK* group
     - commonly-acquired *Staphylococcus aureus* or enterococci in absence of primary focus
   - persistently positive blood culture defined as a micro-organism consistent with infective endocarditis from:
     - blood cultures drawn more than 12 hours apart
     - all three, or majority of four or more blood cultures with first and last drawn at least 1 hour apart.
2. Evidence of endocardial involvement: positive echocardiogram for infective endocarditis.
3. Oscillating intracardiac mass on valve or supporting structure in the path of regurgitant stream or on iatrogenic devices in the absence of an alternative anatomical explanation.
4. Abscess.
5. New partial dehiscence of a prosthetic valve of new valvular regurgitation (worsening or changing of pre-existing murmur not sufficient).

Clinical criteria: minor criteria

1. Predisposing heart condition or i.v. drug use.
2. Fever ≥ 38°C.
3. Vascular phenomena: arterial embolism, septic pulmonary infarcts, mycotic aneurysm, intracranial haemorrhage, Janeway lesions.
4. Immunological phenomena: glomerulonephritis, Osler's nodes, Roth spots.
5. Echocardiogram consistent with infective endocarditis but not meeting major criteria, or serological evidence of active infection with organism consistent with infective endocarditis.

* HACEK: *Haemophilus, Actinobacillus, Cardiobacterium, Eikinella* and *Kingella* spp.

THERAPY

- Give antibiotics [A] once there is a positive blood culture, [C] or sooner if endocarditis is strongly suspected. [A]
  - Give combination therapy (commonly a broad-spectrum penicillin plus an aminoglycoside) [C] intravenously for at least 2 weeks [C] and probably longer, [D] e.g. benzylpenicillin 1200 mg four times a day and gentamicin 80 mg twice a day for 4 weeks.

Commonest organisms in infective endocarditis [B]

- *Streptococcus viridans*
- *Staphylococcus aureus*
- other streptococci
- Enterococci
- HACEK group.

- Ask for a cardiothoracic surgical opinion if any of the following is present: [B]
  - left ventricular failure
  - recurrent embolism
  - uncontrolled infection.

REVIEW

Advise patients to have antibiotic prophylaxis for dental, medical or surgical procedures. [A]

Outcomes

- Around one in 10 with infective endocarditis dies in hospital. [B] The risk is increased with prosthetic valves, [B] embolic events [B] or neurological complications. [C]
- Half will require surgery. [B]
- A quarter develop neurological complications. [A]
- One in seven has an embolic event. [B]

Expires July 2003   Guideline: Chris Ball, Carl Hennigan, Sumit Dhingra
CATs: Chris Ball, Carl Hennigan, Sumit Dhingra, Clare Wotton

28
INFLAMMATORY BOWEL DISEASE

SYMPTOMS AND SIGNS

First attack of colitis (prolonged bloody diarrhoea)
Ask about:
- speed of onset, particularly:
  + an insidious one [C]
- number of bowel movements per day at onset [C]

> **Note**
> Fewer than four bowel movements a day makes inflammatory bowel disease more likely. [C]

The following make inflammatory bowel disease less likely:
- any fever [C]
- any recent travel abroad [C]
- severe abdominal pain [C]
- vomiting. [C]

> **Common causes of colitis include:** [C]
> - inflammatory bowel disease
> - infectious colitis:
>   - bacterial
>   - amoebic
> - pseudomembranous colitis.
>
> Think about: [D]
> - diverticular disease
> - bowel cancer
> - ischaemic colitis
> - radiation colitis
> - ileocaecal TB.

Look for:
+ macroscopically bloody stool [C]
- dehydration or hypovolaemia
- septicaemia/septic shock
- evidence of perforation.

Known ulcerative colitis
Ask patients about:
- number of bowel motions per day, and whether there was any blood. [C]

Truelove criteria

Severe disease:

- six or more motions a day with macroscopic blood
- fever > 37.8° C on 2 out of 4 days
- pulse > 90 beats per minute
- anaemia < 75% predicted
- ESR > 30 mm/h.

Moderate:

- not severe or mild.

Mild:

- fewer than four motions a days with no more than small amounts of macroscopic blood
- no fever
- pulse < 90 beats per minute
- anaemia not severe
- ESR < 30 mm/h.

Look for: [C]

- tachycardia
- fever
- dehydration or hypovolaemia
- septicaemia/septic shock
- evidence of perforation
- anaemia
- raised ESR.

Known Crohn's disease

Ask about: [C]

- general well-being in last 24 hours
- any abdominal pain in last 24 hours
- the number of liquid stools per day.

Look for: [C]

- an abdominal mass
- any systemic complications
- weight loss > 2.5 kg
- lower GI bleeding
- anal fissures or abscesses
- dehydration or hypovolaemia
- septicaemia/septic shock
- evidence of perforation.

Use the following clinical prediction rule to help determine your patient's risk of a current relapse. [C]

Clinical feature	Score
General well-being in last 24 hours	
• very well	0
• slightly below par	1
• poor	2
• very poor	3
• terrible	4
Abdominal pain in last 24 hours	
• none	0
• mild	1
• moderate	2
• severe	3
Number of liquid stools per day	1 point per episode
Abdominal mass	
• none	0
• dubious	1
• definite	2
• definite and tender	3
Systemic complications	score 1 per item
• arthralgia	
• uveitis	
• erythema nodosum	
• aphthous ulcers	
• pyoderma gangrenosum	
• anal fissure	
• new fistula	
• abscess	

Score	Risk of Crohn's relapse
≥ 7	95%
4 to 6	60%
≤ 3	2%

INVESTIGATIONS

- Blood count. [C]
- ESR. [C]
- Group & save/cross-match blood. [D]
- U&E, creatinine. [D]
- CRP. [B]
- Glucose. [D]
- Calcium, magnesium. [D]

- Liver function tests. [B]
- Stool culture and microscopy. [D]
- *Clostridium difficile* toxin assay. [D]
- Erect chest X-ray. [D]
- Abdominal X-ray.

Abdominal X-ray
Look for:
- extent of colitis: extent of faecal residue, evidence of mucosal ulceration and alteration of haustral pattern [C]
- presence of three or more loops of gas-filled small bowel indicating small bowel distension. [C]

Consider:
± arranging for colonoscopy [C] with biopsies [D]

Note
- 1% of patients with acute colitis suffer toxic dilation following colonoscopy. [C]
- Barium follow-through studies are unhelpful in diagnosing IBD. [C]

- an air enema [B] (if ulcerative colitis exacerbation).

Air enema
Look for:
- severe changes: an irregular mucosal contour, > 2 mm deep ulceration or ulceration undermining the mucosa (suggesting deep ulceration).

Consider the following in a first episode of colitis (if inflammatory bowel disease suspected):
+ p-ANCA [C]
- abdominal ultrasound scan [B]
− white cell scanning. [C]

Abdominal ultrasound scan
A normal scan makes Crohn's disease less likely. [B]

THERAPY

- Resuscitate your patient and give blood if required. [A]
- Give steroids, [A] e.g.:
  - hydrocortisone 200 mg i.v. three times daily
  - prednisolone 30 mg daily by mouth.

Use rectal steroids for mild to moderate distal ulcerative colitis. [A]

- Give 5-aminosalicylates, [A] e.g. mesalazine 800 mg three times a day. For patients with distal ulcerative colitis, add[A] rectal 5-aminosalicylates, [A] e.g. mesalazine enema 1 g daily.

> **5-aminosalicylates**
> - Watch out for blood dyscrasias.
> - Warn patients to report: [D]
>   - any unexplained bleeding or bruising
>   - a sore throat, fever or malaise.

- Give antibiotics:
  - ciprofloxacin in ulcerative colitis: [A] 400 mg twice daily by mouth
  - metronidazole in perianal and colonic Crohn's disease: [A] 500 mg i.v. three times a day.
- Consider using nicotine patches for patients with ulcerative colitis who have relapsed on therapy. [A]

Ask for a surgical opinion if there are any of the following: [D]
- toxic megacolon
- free perforation of the colon
- massive haemorrhage
- septicaemia
- severe metabolic disturbance or secondary organ failure
- failure to improve on medical therapy.

For active disease that fails to respond to steroids, consider:
- antimetabolites: [A] azathioprine, methotrexate, 6-mercaptopurine

> **Note**
> - Side-effects are common – careful monitoring is required. [A]
> - Look for:
>   - nausea
>   - leukopenia
>   - infection
>   - abnormal liver function tests
>   - pancreatitis.

- cyclosporin [A]
- infliximab [A] for Crohn's disease, particularly with chronic abdominal or anal fistulae. [A]

REVIEW

- Monitor:
  - vital signs, [C] particularly fever and tachycardia
  - number of stools passed per day [B]

- blood count [C]
- inflammatory markers [B]
- urea and electrolytes [D]
- plain abdominal film for small bowel distension. [C]

Note

Continued frequent diarrhoea and elevated inflammatory markers increase the risk of colectomy. [B]

- Look for evidence of toxic megacolon. [C]

Toxic megacolon
- Look for: [C]
  - abdominal distension
  - localized or generalized peritonitis
  - fever > 38°C
  - tachycardia > 120 beats/minute
  - leukocytosis > 11×10^9/L
  - small bowel distension on plain abdominal X-ray. [C]
- 10% of patients with acute ulcerative colitis develop toxic dilation compared with 2% of patients with acute Crohn's disease. [C]
- One in six dies. [C]

- Withdraw steroids gradually once clinical symptoms and inflammatory markers are improving. [A]

Ulcerative colitis:

Give 5-aminosalicylates, preferably sulfasalazine, [A] as tablets (500 mg four times a day) and enemas (3 g at night, retained for at least 1 hour) on recovery. [A]

Crohn's disease:

- Advise patients to stop smoking. [C]
- Give fish oil on recovery. [A]

For patients with frequent relapses, [D] give:
- oral budesonide 6 mg daily [B]
- azathioprine 2 mg/kg daily. [A]

Following surgery, give:
- mesalamine [A] 400 to 800 mg three times a day
- cimetidine 400 mg four times a day for extensive ileal resection. [A]

Outcomes
- One in three patients with acute colitis requires a colectomy. [B]
- Relapses and subsequent surgery are common following discharge. [B]
- Systemic manifestations are uncommon – the commonest are joint problems. [B]
- Cancer is uncommon. [C]

29
MENINGITIS

SYMPTOMS AND SIGNS

Ask about:
- fever [B]
- nausea and vomiting [A]
- headache [B]
- neck stiffness [B]
- photophobia. [D]

> **Think about other causes of headache:** [D]
> - subarachnoid haemorrhage
> - encephalitis
> - cerebral abscess
> - other causes of raised intracranial pressure
> - migraine.

Look for:
- fever [B]
+ neck stiffness [B]
- altered mental state [B]
- photophobia [D]
- rash
+ Kernig's sign (positive if your patient's headache worsens on flexing the legs at the hip and extending them at the knees) [B]
- jolt accentuation (positive if your patient's headache worsens on rotating the head 2 or 3 times) [A]
- raised intracranial pressure
  - papilloedema
  - absence of retinal vein pulsation.

> **Common causes of meningitis include:** [D]
> - *Neisseria meningitidis*
> - *Streptococcus pneumoniae*
> - Gram-negative bacilli.
>
> Remember:
> - *Listeria monocytogenes*
> - *Haemophilus influenzae*
> - tuberculosis
> - *Cryptococcus*
> - viral infection (Coxsackie, ECHO virus, mumps, polio).

INVESTIGATIONS

- Blood count. [D]
- Clotting studies. [D]
- U&E, creatinine. [A]
- Glucose. [D]
- Blood cultures. [A]
- Chest X-ray. [D]
- Throat swab. [D]
- Lumbar puncture: [A]
  - send CSF for:
    - Gram stain and cell count [A]
    - culture [A]
    - glucose and protein. [C]

For interpretation of results, see Table 29.1.

Lumbar puncture
- Consider arranging a CT brain scan before performing the lumbar puncture, particularly if there is: [A]
  - papilloedema
  - focal neurological signs
  - altered mental state.
- Use a narrow-gauge, non-cutting needle, [A] through a bleb of local anaesthetic. [C]
- Replace the stylet before withdrawing the needle. [A]
- There is no clear benefit from bedrest post-lumbar puncture – it does not reduce lumbar-puncture headache. [D]

Table 29.1 Typical cerebrospinal fluid results [D]

	Cell count /m³	Main cell type	Protein g/dl	CSF: blood glucose
Bacterial	> 1000	Polymorphs	> 1.5	< 50%
Viral	< 500	Lymphocytes	0.5 to 1	> 50%
TB	< 500	Lymphocytes	1 to 5	< 50%
Fungal	< 150	Lymphocytes	0.5 to 1	< 50%

Consider:

- sending for PCR if viral meningitis suspected. [C]
- using a leukocyte-esterase reagent dipstick to detect bacterial meningitis. [B]

Note
A positive or trace reading on leukocyte-esterase dipstick makes bacterial meningitis more likely. [B]

THERAPY

- Resuscitate and seek help if needed.
- Give antibiotics [A] once meningitis is suspected, [D] e.g. ceftriaxone 2 to 4 g i.v. daily.

  Consider giving:
  - ampicillin 500 mg i.v. to elderly patients [D]
  - aciclovir 10 mg/kg i.v. over 1 hour every 8 hours if herpes simplex encephalitis is a possibility.

- Give analgesia. [A]
- Treat sepsis – patients may require: [D]
  - central venous access
  - a urinary catether
  - transfer to an intensive care unit.

REVIEW

Contact your local communicable disease team to arrange chemoprophylaxis for household contact of patients with *Neisseria meningitidis* meningitis.

Chemoprophylaxis
Give a single dose of oral rifampicin 600 mg twice daily for 2 days [A] or ceftriaxone 250 mg i.m. once. [A]

Outcomes
- Around a quarter of patients with bacterial meningitis die, [B] though only one in fifteen with meningococcal meningitis dies.
- A quarter develop seizures, [B] and long-term neurological problems are common, with one in nine having severe disability. [C]
- Viral meningitis is less severe, with only one in nine having a serious illness. [C]

Expires July 2003   Guideline: Bob Phillips, Chris Ball
                        CATs: Bob Phillips, Chris Ball, Clare Wotton

30
MYOCARDIAL INFARCTION

SYMPTOMS AND SIGNS

Myocardial infarction
Defined as two of:
- chest pain lasting 20 minutes or more
- a characteristic rise and fall of cardiac enzymes
- characteristic ECG changes.

Ask about:
- the pain, specifically:
  - its position, [B] looking for:
    + chest or left arm pain [B]
  - its duration, [A] looking for:
    + chest pain which started ≥ 48 hours ago [A]
    + constant pain [B]
  - its nature, [A] looking for:
    + pressure [A]
    − no sharp or stabbing pain [A]
    − no pleuritic pain [A]
    − no positional pain [A]
  - any radiation [A] particularly to:
    + both arms [B]
    + the right shoulder [B]
    + the left arm [B]
  + any similarity to previous infarcts or angina attacks [A]
  - any exacerbating or relieving factors, [B] particularly:
    + pain brought on by exertion
    + pain relieved by nitrates or rest

Other common causes of chest pain include: [C]
- angina
- pulmonary embolism
- chest infection
- musculoskeletal pain
- pericarditis.

Rarer causes include: [D]
- aortic dissection
- oesophageal spasm
- oesophageal rupture

> - abdominal pain
>   - gallstones
>   - gastritis
> - herpes zoster.

+ any nausea or vomiting [A]
+ any sweating [B]
■ a history of:
   + angina or MI [A]
   + heart failure [A]
   + an acute respiratory infection in the previous 10 days [B]
■ cardiovascular risk factors:
   ■ hypertension [A]
   ■ smoking [B]
   ■ diabetes mellitus [A]
   ■ elevated total cholesterol or triglycerides [A]

Note
Cardiovascular risk factors are not very helpful at diagnosing a myocardial infarction, but increase the risk of complications and death. [B]

■ usual levels of activity [A]
■ a parental history of angina or MI before the age of 60. [A]

Look for:
+ sweating [B]
+ hypotension [B]
■ Kussmaul's sign (JVP rising during quiet inspiration) [C]

Note
Kussmaul's sign makes right ventricular infarction more likely in patients with an inferior MI. [C]

+ a third [B] or fourth heart sound [C]
− chest pain that is reproduced on palpation [A]
+ pulmonary crackles. [A]

INVESTIGATIONS

■ Blood count. [B]

Note
A high leukocyte count makes a myocardial infarction more likely. [B]

- U&E, creatinine. [D]
- Glucose. [A]
- Serial cardiac enzymes:
    - ± CK-MB over 24 hours [C]
    - ± troponin T [C]
    - ± creatinine kinase [B] over 48 hours with:
        - **+** lactate dehydrogenase. [A]

Note
- An early CK-MB rise diagnoses a myocardial infarction and normal levels at 20 hours rule it out. [C]
- A normal troponin T or troponin I at 20 hours makes an infarct unlikely. [C]
- Elevated creatinine kinase levels [B] or an elevated myoglobin[C] diagnoses an infarct.
- CK, AST or LDH taken on presentation cannot safely diagnose or exclude an infarct. [A]

- Lipid levels. [A]
- ± 12-lead ECG, [A] followed by serial ECGs. [B]
- Chest X-ray. [A]

ECG
- Look for features suggesting cardiac ischaemia:
    - any ST elevation in two or more leads [A]
    - any ST depression [B]
    - any Q waves [A]
    - any T wave inversion [B]
    - any conduction defect. [B]
- These are more significant if present in two or more leads, or not known to be old.
- A normal ECG makes life-threatening complications unlikely. [C]

Use the clinical prediction rule given in Table 12.1 (p. 50) to rank your patient for risk of a myocardial infarction. [A]

THERAPY

- Give oxygen. [D]
- Give analgesia: [A]
    - nitrous oxide with oxygen [B]
    - opiate analgesia, [A] e.g. diamorphine 1 mg/min i.v. until pain relieved (up to 10 mg)
- Metoclopramide [D] 10 mg i.v. over 1 to 2 min.

- Give aspirin [A] 300 mg orally, [D] then 75 mg daily. [A] Alternatives include:
  - clopidogrel [A] 525 mg daily, then 75 mg daily.

For patients with pain that started within 12 hours and any of:
  - > 2 mm ST elevation in two adjacent limb leads
  - > 1 mm ST elevation in two adjacent chest leads
  - new LBBB:

- Offer primary angioplasty if available. [A]
- Otherwise give thrombolysis [A] as soon as possible [A] if there are no contraindications.

Contraindications to thrombolysis
- active bleeding [A]
- recent surgery or trauma [C]
- recent stroke [A]
- active peptic ulcer disease [D]
- evidence of aortic dissection. [D]

Ideally use reteplase [A] or tPA (alteplase), [A] followed by a heparin infusion for 24 hours, particularly for:
- older patients [A]
- patients with an anterior MI [A]
- patients who have received streptokinase or anistreplase longer than 4 days ago. [D]

Otherwise use streptokinase. [A]

Thrombolysis
- Reteplase: 10 units over 1 to 2 minutes, followed by another 10 units 30 minutes later.
- tPA (alteplase): 15 mg i.v. over 1 to 2 minutes, followed by 50 mg i.v. over 30 minutes, then 35 mg over 60 minutes (max 1.5 mg/kg in patients > 65 kg).
- Streptokinase: 1.5 million units in 100 ml 0.9% saline, given over 1 hour.

Heparin
- Add 25 000 units heparin to 50 ml 0.9% saline.
- Give a bolus of 5000 units, then infuse at 1000 units/hr (2 ml/h).
- Check aPTT 6 hours later. Aim for an aPTT ratio 1.5 to 2.5.

See Chapter 19 for more details on heparin dosing.

Note
- One in eight patients has a moderate or severe bleed after thrombolysis. [B]
- 1% have a stroke. [B]

Give patients with an admission glucose > 11.0 mmol/L: [A]
- an insulin–glucose infusion for 24 hours, followed by subcutaneous insulin four times daily for at least 3 months.

An insulin infusion regimen
Add 50 units of actrapid (soluble) insulin to 50 ml of 0.9% saline. Infuse using the following sliding scale.

Glucose mmol/L	Infusion rate units/hr
0 to 4	0.5 and 10% or 20% glucose infusion
4 to 8	1
8 to 12	2
12 to 16	3
16 to 20	4
>20	6 and call doctor

The regimen may need to be adjusted depending on your patient's response.

Start:
- a beta-blocker [A] once thrombolysis is completed, [A] e.g. metoprolol 25 mg three times a day, or atenolol 50 mg daily.
- an ACE inhibitor [A] within 36 hours, particularly for patients with:
  - a reduced LV ejection fraction (< 40%), [A] unless patients have cardiogenic shock or a systolic blood pressure < 100 mmHg [C]
  - one other cardiovascular risk factor (hypertension, hypercholesterolaemia, low HDL levels, smoking or documented microalbuminuria). [A]

ACE inhibitors
- Monitor the blood pressure for the first dose. [D]
- Increase the dose if patients tolerate it.
- Typical doses:
  - enalapril 2.5 to 5 mg daily initially, increasing to 10 to 20 mg daily.
  - perindopril 1 mg daily initially increasing to 4 to 8 mg daily.
  - ramipril 1.25 mg daily initially increasing to 5 mg daily. [A]
- Monitor the renal function. [A]

Consider:
- anticoagulating patients with an anterior MI who do not receive thrombolysis [A]
- giving an LMWH long-term [A]
- amiodarone. [A]

Amiodarone

Loading dose:
- intravenous:
  - preferably via a central line
  - Give 300 mg (5 mg/kg) in 250 ml 5.0% glucose over 1 hour, followed by 900 mg over 24 hours.

- oral:
  - Give 200 mg every 8 hours for 1 week, then 200 mg every 12 hours for 1 week, then start maintenance therapy.

Maintenance dose:
- Patients should be given a total loading dose of 4200 mg before starting on maintenance therapy. [D]
- Give 100 to 200 mg daily.

REVIEW

- Observe patients for at least 5 days. [D]
- Repeat cardiac enzymes [A] and ECGs [A] daily for at least 2 days. [D]

Ask about:
- further chest pain [A]
- dyspnoea [A]
- palpitations. [A]

Angina
See Chapter 6 for more information.

Look for: [B]
- Arrhythmias, particularly AV block, VF or sustained VT:
  - Give amiodarone to patients with ventricular arrhythmias. [A]
  - Avoid using:
    - class Ic anti-arrhythmic agents [A]
    - sotalol. [A]

Arrhythmias
- One in five has an episode of bradycardia within 4 hours, but many settle, with only a tenth having symptoms after this time. [B] Bradycardia is commoner in inferior MI. [A]

See Chapters 8 (bradyarrhythmias) and 40 (tachycardias) for more information.

- New murmurs or a pericardial rub, particular evidence of: [B]
  - mitral regurgitation [B]
  - ventricular septal rupture [B]
  - ventricular aneurysms. [B]

> **Note**
> - One in 14 develops mitral regurgitation. [B]
> - One in 50 develops ventricular rupture [B] – half will die. [B]

Give NSAIDs is there is evidence of pericarditis. [C]
Start anticoagulation if a ventricular aneurysm is present. [A]

- Signs of heart failure, [B] particularly cardiogenic shock. [A]

Heart failure	
Killip class [C]	Signs
I	No clinical signs of heart failure
II	Crackles, S_3 gallop and elevated JVP
III	Frank pulmonary oedema
IV	Cardiogenic shock, hypotension (systolic BP < 90 mmHg), evidence of peripheral vasoconstriction (oliguria, cyanosis, sweating)

> **Note**
> One in 14 develops cardiogenic shock [A] – half will die. [A]
>
> See Chapter 21 for more information on congestive heart failure.

Provide cardiac rehabilitation involving: [A]
- a structured exercise programme [A]
- psychosocial interventions [A] – encourage patients to be realistic about their illness. [C]

Target cardiac risk factors:
- Encourage patients to stop smoking [A] and ask nurses [A] and other staff [A] to provide further advice.
  Offer:
  - nicotine patches [A] or gum [A]
  - buproprion. [A]
- Treat hypertension. [A]
- Optimize diabetes control. [A]
- Lower cholesterol levels [A] even for patients with average levels (cholesterol 4.0 to 6.2 mmol/L) [A] using:
  - diet modification. [A] Encourage patients to eat a Mediterranean-style diet [A]

> **Dietary advice**
> - Eat more bread, more root and green vegetables, fish, and oats. [A]
> - Eat less meat – replace beef, lamb, pork with poultry.
> - Have no day without fruit.
> - Replace butter and cream with margarine, rapeseed and olive oils.
> - Eat more soy protein. [B]

- a statin [A]

Statins
Start at a low dose and increase to the maximum tolerated e.g.: [D]
- atorvastatin 40 mg at night
- pravastatin 40 mg at night
- simvastatin 40 mg at night.

- gemfibrozil 600 mg twice daily for patients with low HDL levels. [A]

Consider giving patients:
- n-3 polyunsaturated fatty acid supplements [A]
- vitamin E supplements [A] 400 mg daily.

Stress-testing
Perform stress-testing before discharge or as an outpatient [D] using the guide in Chapter 6 (page 27).

Outcomes
- One in 30 dies within 10 days, [A] rising to one in eight at 2 years, [B] and 60% at 10 years. [B]
- One in 40 has another MI within a year [A] – a third have another MI within 10 years. [B]
- One in nine develops angina within a year. [A]
- A third of patients with ventricular aneurysms die within 5 years. [B]
- One in 18 has an episode of VF within 6 months – one in five dies. [B]

31
PLEURAL EFFUSIONS

SYMPTOMS AND SIGNS

Ask about:
+ weight loss [C]
+ fever [C]
■ previous diagnoses. [D]

Note
Weight loss > 4.5 kg, or fever > 38° C makes malignancy or granulomatous disease more likely. [C]

Look for:
■ reduced expansion [D]
■ stony dullness on percussion [D]
■ diminished breath sounds
■ change in dullness on auscultatory percussion. [B]

Auscultatory percussion [B]
• Ask your patient to sit upright or stand for 5 minutes to allow any free pleural fluid to drain to the lung base.
• Place the stethoscope diaphragm 3 cm below the 12th rib in the midclavicular line.
• Percuss directly with your free hand (by finger flicking or with the pulp of a finger) along three or more parallel lines from the apex of each hemithorax perpendicularly down towards the base.
• Pleural effusions can be confirmed by asking a patient to lean to one side and then reassess the fluid level to see whether it has shifted.

Common causes include: [B]
Transudates:
• congestive heart failure
• liver cirrhosis
• nephrotic syndrome
• hypoalbuminaemia.

Exudates:
• malignant effusions
• parapneumonic effusions
• tuberculosis

- pulmonary embolism
- collagen vascular disease
- trauma
- pancreatitis.

INVESTIGATIONS

Arrange for a chest X-ray [C] or ultrasound scan. [C]

Chest X-ray
A large effusion (> half a hemithorax) increases the risk of malignancy or TB. [C]

Perform thoracentesis. [C]

Thoracentesis
- Perform under ultrasound guidance [A], otherwise use a 20 G needle and syringe. [A]
- Watch out for any subsequent pneumothorax. [C]

Look at the fluid collected [C] and send it for: [C]
- biochemistry:
  - protein [C]
  - glucose [B]
  - LDH [B]
  - pH [B]
- cytology [C]
- microscopy and culture of fluid.

If indicated, consider:
- amylase (suspected pancreatitis or oesophageal rupture) [C]
- triglycerides [C] (suspected chylous fluid)
- tumour markers
  - carcinoembryonic antigen (CEA) [C]
  - complement (C_3, C_4) [C]
  - α1-antitrypsin [C]
- antinuclear antibodies [C] (suspected SLE)
- interferon-gamma (positive if > 140 pg/ml) [C] (suspected TB)
- adenosine deaminase (positive if > 45 U/l) [B] (suspected TB).

Consider taking the following blood tests:
- blood count [D]
- urea and electrolytes [D]
- glucose [C]
- protein [B]
- liver function tests [B]

- albumin [B]
- calcium [D]
- tumour markers. [C]

If there is still no clear diagnosis, consider: [C]
- repeating the thoracentesis [D]
- needle biopsy [C]
- spiral CT, lung scan (or pulmonary angiography if neither available) [D]
- bronchoscopy. [C]

followed by thoracoscopy [C] if required.

THERAPY

Malignancy

Insert a chest drain [A] and perform pleurodesis in recurrent cases. [A]

Perform pleurodesis once [D] after the chest tube is draining < 150 ml of fluid per day [A] and a chest X-ray shows [B] no remaining fluid. [D]

Options include:
- surgical pleurodesis under thoracoscopy [D] using talc [B]
- medical pleurodesis using any of the following for pleurodesis:
  - tetracycline [B] and bleomycin [A]
  - doxycycline [B]
  - minocycline [B]
  - mepacrine. [A]

Pleurodesis using tetracycline and bleomycin
- Make up tetracycline 1.5 g freshly dissolved in 40 ml 0.9% saline and 20 ml 1% lignocaine.
- Make up bleomycin 1 unit/kg to a max of 60 units in 50 ml of normal saline.
- Pain and fever are common after pleurodesis [B] so give prophylactic analgesia.
- Instil tetracycline and bleomycin
- Flush tube with 30 to 50 ml 0.9% saline. Then clamp the drain.
- Ask the patient to lie 15 minutes affected side up, 15 minutes affected side down, 15 minutes prone, then 15 minutes supine. [D]
- Allow to drain until < 100 ml draining over 24 hours, then remove chest drain. [D]
- Consider injecting intrapleural bupivacaine to reduce pain for up to 4 hours. [A]

Note
Rotating a patient during medical pleurodesis has no clear effect on the long-term success of the procedure. [D]

Parapneumonic effusion

Drain a parapneumonic effusion if it is purulent or loculated: [D]

- Insert a chest drain. [A]
- Instil streptokinase [A] 250 000 units in 100 ml 0.9% saline daily or urokinase [D] 100 000 units in 100 ml 0.9% saline daily into the chest drain and clamp for 3 hours.

Refer patients for surgery if drainage is unsuccessful. [D]

Tuberculosis

- Give antituberculous chemotherapy.
- If TB is prevalent consider empiric treatment in patients where no clear cause can be found. [D]
- Insert a chest drain. [D]

REVIEW

Watch out for complications from the chest drain. [B]

Chest drain complications

Common complications include: [B]

- subcutaneous emphysema
- air leak lasting more than 7 days.

Less common problems include:

- infection [B]
- tube slippage [B]
- re-expansion pulmonary oedema. [B]

Outcomes

- Half of patients with malignant effusions have a recurrence within 6 months. [B] 90% are dead within 2 years. [B]
- If no cause can be found, despite extensive investigation, only a sixth will relapse. [C]

Expires July 2003   Guideline: Chris Ball
CATs: Chris Ball, Clare Wotton, Don Stanley

32
COMMUNITY-ACQUIRED PNEUMONIA

SYMPTOMS AND SIGNS

Ask about:
- the duration of illness [C]
- any recent diarrhoea [C]
- pleuritic chest pains [B]
- chills [B]
- other medical problems, particularly:
  - asthma [A] or other lung disease [C]
  - + dementia [A]
  - + any immunosuppression [A]
  - cancer
  - heart failure
  - liver disease
  - cerebrovascular disease
  - renal disease
- any pets. [D]

> **Note**
> - Age < 40, and a prodromal illness longer than 9 days favours *Mycoplasma* infection. [C]
> - A history of diarrhoea makes *Legionella* pneumonia more likely. [C]

> **Other causes of dyspnoea include:** [B]
> - asthma
> - heart failure
> - COPD
> - arrhythmias
> - interstitial lung disease
> - anaemia
> - lung cancer [D]
> - pulmonary embolism.

Look for:
- altered mental state [A]
- bloody sputum [A]
- cough [A]
- fever [A]
- respiratory rate > 30 per minute [A]
- tachycardia [A]
- + asymmetric respiration. [A]

> **Note**
> - Bloody sputum makes pneumonococcal pneumonia more likely. [C]
> - No fever, tachycardia or tachypnoea makes pneumonia less likely.

Listen for:
+ dullness on percussion [A]
+ decreased breath sounds [A]
+ bronchial breathing [A]
+ crackles [A]
+ aegophony. [A]

> **Risk of pulmonary infiltrate on chest X-ray** [A]
> Score one point for: [A]
> - absence of asthma
> - temperature > 37.8°C
> - pulse > 100 beats/min
> - crackles
> - decreased breath sounds.
>
> | Score | Risk of pneumonia |
> | --- | --- |
> | 4 or 5 | High (60%) |
> | 2 or 3 | Moderate (13%) |
> | 0 or 1 | Low (3%) |

INVESTIGATIONS

■ Pulse oximetry. [C]
+ Blood count. [C]
■ U&E, creatinine. [A]
■ Glucose. [A]
■ Creatine kinase. [C]

> **Note**
> A raised creatine kinase makes *Legionella* pneumonia more likely. [C]

■ Blood cultures. [C]
■ Sputum Gram stain, and culture. [D]
■ Serology if atypical organisms suspected: [A]
  ■ *Mycoplasma pneumoniae*
  ■ *Legionella pneumophila*
  ■ *Chlamydia psittaci*
  ■ influenza A and B
  ■ *Coxiella burnetii*.
■ Urine for *Legionella* antigen. [C]
■ Arterial blood gas. [A]
■ Chest X-ray. [A]

Chest X-ray changes
Look for:
- a lobar infiltrate [C] – this makes pneumococcal pneumonia more likely
- pleural effusion. [A]

Consider:
- a bronchoalveolar lavage [A] if the diagnosis remains uncertain.

THERAPY

- Give oxygen to hypoxic patients. [A]

- Give antibiotics [A] intravenously to complicated cases. Uncomplicated cases can have oral antibiotics. [A]

Complicated pneumonias include:
- acute confusion
- immunocompromised
- critically ill
- requiring inotropic or respiratory support
- septicaemia
- unable to tolerate oral medication
- pregnant or lactating.

Common causes include: [D]
- *Streptococcus pneumoniae*
- *Mycoplasma pneumoniae*
Less common causes include:
- Influenza A virus
- *Haemophilus influenzae*
- *Chlamydia psittaci*
- *Legionella pneumophila*
- *Coxiella burnetii*
- *Staphylococcus aureus*.

- Give amoxicillin [D] 500 mg every 8 hours, [D] with erythromycin 500 mg every 6 hours if an atypical pneumonia is possible. [D]
- Give elderly patients any of:
  - a second or third generation cephalosporin with a macrolide, [B] e.g. cefuroxime 1.5 g every 8 hours with erythromycin 500 mg every 6 hours
  - a fluroquinilone, [B] e.g. ciprofloxacin 400 mg every 12 hours.
- For aspiration pneumonia, add metronidazole 500 mg every 8 hours to cover anaerobes. [D]

- Give analgesia for pleuritic pain, e.g. an NSAID.

- Consider transferring patients with any of the following to the intensive care unit: [D]
  - severe pneumonia
  - severe hypoxia despite high-flow oxygen ($SaO_2 < 90\%$ on $\geq 50\%$ oxygen)
  - exhausted, drowsy or unconscious patient
  - respiratory or cardiac arrest
  - shock.

Consider:
- continuous positive airway pressure (CPAP) for respiratory failure. [A]

Parapneumonic effusion
- Drain a parapneumonic effusion if it is purulent or loculated. [D]
- Insert a chest drain, [A] and instil streptokinase [A] 250 000 units in 20 ml daily or urokinase. [D]
- Refer patients for surgery if drainage is unsuccessful. [D]

REVIEW

- Monitor your patient's response, [C] and repeat investigations if there is no improvement after 72 hours. [D]
- Advise elderly patients or patients with lung disease to have the influenza vaccine. [A]
- Risk of death within 1 month can be assessed from Table 32.1.

Table 32.1   Risk of dying from pneumonia in the next month [A]

Factor	Score
Age	Years for men years − 10 for women
Nursing home resident	+10
Co-existing disease:	
Neoplastic disease	+30
Liver disease	+20
Congestive heart failure	+10
Cerebrovascular disease	+10
Renal disease	+10
Physical findings:	
Altered mental status	+20
Respiratory rate > 30 per minute	+20
Systolic blood pressure < 90 mmHg	+20
Temperature < 35°C or > 40°C	+15
Pulse > 125 beats/minute	+10

(Continued)

Factor	Score
Laboratory and radiographic findings:	
Arterial pH < 7.35	+30
Urea > 11 mmol/L	+20
Sodium < 130 mmol/L	+20
Glucose > 14 mmol/L	+10
Haematocrit < 30%	+10
pO_2 < 8.0 kPa	+10
Pleural effusion	+10

Score	Class	Risk of dying within 30 days
> 130	V	High (27%)
91 to 130	IV	Moderate (9%)
71 to 90	III	Low (0.6%)
< 70	II	Low (0.3%)
Aged < 50 and none of the conditions or physical findings listed	I	Low (0.1%)

Outcomes
- One in seven patients fails to respond to the first antibiotic regimen. [C]
- One in 20 patients dies. [A]

33
SPONTANEOUS PNEUMOTHORAX

SYMPTOMS AND SIGNS

A spontaneous pneumothorax is common in:
- patients with sudden onset dyspnoea and chest pain [C]
- young men. [D]

Ask about:
- previous episodes of spontaneous pneumothorax [B]
- conditions associated with pulmonary fibrosis [B]
- breathlessness [C]
- pleuritic chest pain [C]
- smoking. [C]

Think about other causes of dypsnoea:
- asthma
- heart failure
- COPD
- arrhythmia
- infection
- interstitial lung disease
- anaemia
- pulmonary embolism.

Look for:
- a tall and thin habitus [B]
- reduced expansion [D]
- a hyperresonant percussion note [D]
- reduced or absent breath sounds [D]
- tracheal shift [D]
- features of respiratory failure. [D]

Causes of a spontaneous pneumothorax
- Most cases are idiopathic. [B]
- One in six is due to secondary causes including:
  - bullous emphysema [B]
  - asthma [C]
  - bronchogenic carcinoma [C]
  - TB. [B]

- Remember rarer causes such as:
  - AIDS [B]
  - fibrosing lung diseases – sarcoidosis, histiocytosis, lymphangioleiomyomatosis [B]
  - bronchiectasis [C]
  - Marfan syndrome. [C]

INVESTIGATIONS

- Pulse oximetry. [D]
- Arterial blood gases. [D]
- ± Chest X-ray. [C]

Chest X-rays
- Expiratory films are not clearly better than inspiratory films for diagnosing a pneumothorax. [C]
- Chest X-rays underestimate the size of a pneumothorax compared with a CT scan. [C]

If uncertain, consider:
- A chest CT. [C]

THERAPY

- Give oxygen if hypoxic. [A]

- Treat a tension pneumothorax immediately by:
  - performing a needle thoracotomy, [A] then
  - inserting a chest drain. [A]

Needle thoracotomy [D]
- Insert a 16–18 gauge cannula into the 2nd intercostal space in the midclavicular line.
- Leave the cap off the end.

Chest drains
- Consider injecting intrapleural bupivacaine to reduce pain for up to 4 hours. [A]
- Provide regular analgesia. [D]
- Remove the drain once the lung is fully expanded. [D]
- There is no clear benefit from adding suction to the chest drain. [D]

- Asymptomatic patients with a small collapse can be treated conservatively. [D]

  Otherwise perform:
  - A catheter aspiration. [A]

Catheter aspiration [C]
- Insert a 16–18 gauge catheter under local anaesthetic into the 2nd intercostal space in the midclavicular line.
- Aspirate air through a 3-way tap.
- Aspirate until no more air can be aspirated, the patient becomes uncomfortable or a maximum of 3 litres has been removed.
- Arrange for a chest X-ray.

  - If the chest X-ray following removal of the catheter shows > 90% lung expansion, consider discharging patients with a primary pneumothorax immediately. [C]
  - Advise patients to return if symptoms recur. [D]
- If this fails, insert a thoracic vent. [A]
- If this fails, insert a chest tube. [A]

- Consider surgical pleurectomy for patients with: [B]
  - a prolonged air leak
  - recurrent pneumothorax
  - bilateral pneumothoraces.

REVIEW

For patients treated with a chest drain:
- Watch out for complications. [B]
- Consider pleurodesis with tetracycline [A] or talc via thoracoscopy. [A]

Chest drain complications
Common complications include: [B]
- subcutaneous emphysema
- an air leak lasting more than 7 days.

Less common problems include:
- infection [B]
- tube slippage [B]
- re-expansion pulmonary oedema. [B]

Outcomes
Recurrent spontaneous pneumothoraces are common, [B] particularly in patients requiring chest drains [B] or with pulmonary fibrosis. [B]

Expires July 2005 Guideline: Chris Ball
CATs: Bob Phillips, Clare Wotton, Chris Ball

34
PULMONARY EMBOLISM

SYMPTOMS AND SIGNS

Use the following clinical prediction rule to work out your patient's risk of a pulmonary embolism. [A]

Step one
Ask about risk factors for venous thromboembolism:
- recent immobilization:
  - paralysis of a leg
  - surgery or a fracture of the leg with immobilization within the last 12 weeks
  - recently bedridden for > 3 days within the last 4 weeks.
- Previous venous thromboembolism (objective diagnosis).
- A strong family history of DVT or PE:
  - two or more family members with objectively-proven events
  - a first-degree relative with hereditary thrombophilia.
- Active cancer (on-going treatment, diagnosed within last 6 months or having palliative care).
- Post-partum.

Step two
Score your patient for the following respiratory points:
- dyspnoea or worsening of chronic dyspnoea
- pleuritic chest pain
- chest pain (non-retrosternal and non-pleuritic)
- arterial oxygen saturation < 92% when breathing room air that corrects with 40% O_2
- haemoptysis
- pleural rub.

Step three
Think about alternative diagnoses.

> **Think about other causes of dypsnoea** [B]
> - asthma
> - heart failure
> - COPD
> - arrhythmia
> - infection
> - interstitial lung disease
> - anaemia.

> **Think about other causes of pleuritic chest pain** [A]
> - viral
> - pneumonia
> - chest wall trauma
> - cancer.

Step four

Decide if your patient's symptoms are atypical, typical or severe for pulmonary embolism (see Table 34.1).

Table 34.1   Classification of symptoms

Symptom type	Symptoms
Atypical	Respiratory or cardiac symptoms not meeting criteria for 'typical'
Typical	Two or more respiratory points and any of the following: • heart rate > 90 beats/min • leg symptoms • low-grade fever • results of chest X-ray compatible with PE
Severe	Typical symptoms and all of the following: • syncope • blood pressure < 90 mmHg with heart rate > 100 beats/min • receiving ventilation or needs oxygen flow > 40% Typical symptoms and: • new onset right heart failure (elevated JVP and new S_1, Q_3 and T_3 or RBBB) All of: • syncope • blood pressure < 90 mmHg with heart rate > 100 beats/min • receiving ventilation or needs oxygen flow > 40% • new onset right heart failure (elevated JVP and new S_1, Q_3 and T_3 or RBBB)

Step five

Decide on your patient's risk for a pulmonary embolism (see Table 34.2).

In addition, ask about features that increase the risk of having a pulmonary embolism:

- use of the oral contraceptive pill [B]
- smoking [A]
- hypertension. [A]

Look for:

- obesity (BMI > 29). [A]

Table 34.2 Risk of PE

Symptom type	Low risk (3%)	Medium risk (30%)	High risk (70%)
Atypical	An alternative diagnosis or no other risk factors	No alternative diagnosis and risk factors	
Typical	An alternative diagnosis and no risk factors	Any other combination	
Severe		An alternative diagnosis	No alternative diagnosis

Body mass index

$$BMI = \frac{\text{weight in kg}}{(\text{height in metres})^2}$$

INVESTIGATIONS

- Blood count. [A]
- Clotting. [D]
- Factor V_{Leiden} and other thrombophilia studies if indicated.
- Cardiac enzymes. [D]
- Arterial blood gases. [A]

Note
Arterial blood gases are unhelpful in diagnosing or excluding PE but can help rule out other conditions. [A]

- ECG. [B]

ECG
Look for:
- a new S_1, Q_3, T_3 (S wave in lead I, Q wave in lead III, T wave inversion in lead III)
- new right bundle-branch block.

- Chest X-ray. [A]

Chest X-ray changes
Look for any abnormality, particularly: [A]
- atelectasis or pulmonary parenchymal abnormality
- pleural effusion
- pleural-based opacity
- decreased pulmonary vasculature
- pulmonary oedema.

Consider:
- a D-dimer in low-risk patients. [A]

> **Note**
> A negative D-dimer can help rule out a PE in low-risk cases. [A]

± Arrange for a ventilation–perfusion scan. [A]

Patients with low or intermediate probability scans need further testing, [C] so base further investigations on the following plan [A] (see Table 34.3).

> **Note**
> • Two-thirds of scans are low or intermediate probability. [A]
> • Pre-existing heart or lung disease does not affect the accuracy of the scan, but more patients have non-diagnostic scans. [A]

Table 34.3   V/Q scan and further testing

V/Q scan result	PE probability	Next test	If required	If required
Normal	Low, moderate or high	Ultrasound: • positive: PE • negative: no PE		
Non-high	Low or moderate	Serial ultrasound (days 1, 3, 7, 14): • positive: PE • negative: no PE		
Non-high	High	Ultrasound: • positive: PE • negative: venogram	Venogram: • positive: PE • negative: pulmonary angiography	Angiography: • positive: PE • negative: no PE
High	Low	Ultrasound: • positive: PE • negative: venogram	Venogram: • positive: PE • negative: pulmonary angiography	Angiography: • positive: PE • negative: no PE
High	Moderate or high	PE		

+ Bilateral compression ultrasound of the leg veins. [A]

Ultrasound

Arrange for compression ultrasound scanning of the common femoral, popliteal and distal popliteal veins. The test is positive if any vein is not fully compressible. [A]

+ Venography. [A]

± Pulmonary angiography. [A]

Pulmonary angiography [C]

1% of patients have major complications:

- death
- haematoma requiring blood transfusion
- renal failure requiring dialysis.

Other helpful tests include:

+ capnography. [A] Look for a low waveform area (< 25 mmHg.sec)

+ impedence plethysmography [B]

+ chest helical CT scan [B]

+ chest MRI. [B]

THERAPY

- Give oxygen if hypoxic. [A]
- Give analgesia for pleuritic pain, e.g. an NSAID – ibuprofen 400 mg three times a day.
- Start anticoagulation [A] in all suspected cases [D] using a low-molecular weight heparin. [D]
- Start warfarin [A] as soon as a pulmonary embolism has been demonstrated. [A]
- Stop the oral contraceptive pill or HRT. [D]

Low-molecular weight heparins

- dalteparin 200 units/kg sc daily
- enoxaparin 1 mg/kg sc twice daily
- tinzaparin 175 units/kg sc once daily

Give LMWH [D] for a minimum of 5 days, and continue for 2 days after the INR is within therapeutic range. [D]

See Chapter 19 for more details on LMWH and warfarin dosing.

Consider the following in life-threatening cases: [D]

- thrombolysis [D]
- embolectomy [D]
- mechanolysis. [D]

Thrombolysis
- tPA (alteplase): 10 mg i.v. over 1 to 2 minutes, followed by 90 mg i.v. over 2 hours (max 1.5 mg/kg in patients < 65 kg).
- Streptokinase: 250 000 units in 100 ml 0.9% saline over 30 minutes, then 100 000 units every hour for 12 to 72 hours.

REVIEW

- Monitor INR levels daily until the warfarin dosing is stable. [D]
- Check the platelet count after 5 days. If it is < 150×10^9/L, then repeat the test. If confirmed, treat for heparin-induced thrombocytopenia. [A]
- Continue warfarin:
  - for 6 weeks for transient risk factors, [D] e.g. surgery, trauma
  - for 6 months for permanent risk factors, [A] e.g. cancer, leg paralysis
  - indefinitely:
    - for idiopathic cases [A]
    - for recurrent venous thromboembolism. [A]

Therapeutic ranges

Indication	Target INR
Venous thromboembolism [C]	2.0 to 3.0
Venous thromboembolism when INR 2.0 to 3.0 [D]	3.0 to 4.5

Outcomes
- Less than 10% of patients have a recurrent PE within a year. [A]
- A quarter are dead within a year; [B] often suddenly, [A] particularly with cancer, heart failure and chronic lung disease. [A]

35
ACUTE RENAL FAILURE

SYMPTOMS AND SIGNS

Acute renal failure
- oliguria: urine output < 400 ml/day
- rapid (hours to weeks) decline in glomerular function rate manifest by increasing urea and creatinine

Ask about: [D]
- systemic diseases: diabetes, vascular disease
- known renal disease and previous renal function tests
- recent systemic disturbances: MI, GI bleeding, recent surgery
- medication, particularly:
  - ACE inhibitors, NSAIDs, diuretics, radiocontrast, aminoglycosides and other antibiotics.

Look for evidence of: [D]
- volume contraction:
  - **+** sunken eyes [B]
  - **+** dry axillae [B]
  - **+** dry nose or mouth mucous membranes [B]
  - **±** longitudinal tongue furrows [B]
  - **±** a low jugular venous pressure [A]

- volume overload:
  - **+** a high jugular venous pressure [A]
  - pulmonary oedema or peripheral oedema [D]

- outflow obstruction
- infection
- joint or skin problems

- multi-organ failure:
  - hypotension despite resuscitation
  - hypoxia despite 40% oxygen
  - metabolic acidosis.

Causes of acute renal failure
Pre-renal causes:
- cardiogenic shock: e.g. hypotension from MI, heart failure
- hypovolaemia: e.g. dehydration, haemorrhage, surgery
- sepsis
- hepatorenal syndrome
- rhabdomyolysis
- HUS, TTP.

Renal causes:
- acute tubular necrosis due to ischaemia: i.e. any pre-renal cause if sufficiently severe or prolonged
- acute tubular necrosis due to drugs or toxins: e.g. aminoglycosides, contrast media
- acute interstitial nephritis
- inflammatory:
  - vasculitis
  - glomerulonephritis
  - scleroderma
  - Goodpasture's syndrome
- vascular:
  - atheroemboli
  - thrombosis
- other causes:
  - myeloma
  - malignant hypertension
  - amyloid.

Post-renal causes:
- obstruction: e.g. stones, prostate, tumour.

The commonest causes are: [C]
- hypotension
- multifactorial
- dehydration
- sepsis
- drugs or contrast.

INVESTIGATIONS

- Blood count [D] and film.
- U&E, creatinine. [A]
- Glucose. [D]

Calculate
- **urea: creatinine ratio:**
  A ratio > 0.1 makes pre-renal failure more likely.

- **estimated creatinine clearance:**
  (ml/min)

  $$\frac{(140 - age) \times weight\ (kg)}{Cr\ (\mu mol/L)}$$

  Multiply by 1.2 for men.

- Normal CrCl ~ 100 ml/min.
- This formula is derived for steady state use (not the case in ARF), but can provide an idea of the severity of the problem.
- If the creatinine is rising, the true clearance will be lower than that calculated.

Consider:
- arterial blood gas, pH [D]
- ECG [D]
- chest X-ray. [D]

If there is no clear cause, consider: [D]
- ESR, CRP
- calcium
- creatine kinase
- blood cultures

- inflammatory screen:
  - autoantibodies: ANA, anti-dsDNA, ANCA, anti-GBM
  - complement
  - cryoglobulins
  - immunoglobulins

- serum and urine electrophoresis

- insert a urethral catheter [A] to exclude lower urinary tract obstruction:
  - record the urine output [D]
  - perform a dipstick and look for:
    - protein [B]
    - leukocytes [B]
    - haemoglobin [B]

Note
Absence of blood or protein on urine dipstick makes glomerular disease less likely. [B]

Send for:
- microscopy – look for comments on:
  - red blood cell shape [B]
  - lymphocytes [B]
  - eosinophils [C]
  - casts [B]

Urine microscopy
Glomerular disease
Look for:
± dysmorphic red blood cells [B]
± absence of haem-granular casts. [B]

Interstitial nephritis
Look for:
± eosinophils [C]
± lymphocytes [B]
± haem-granular casts. [B]

■ culture [D]

■ biochemistry, if trying to distinguish acute tubular necrosis from pre-renal causes:
   ■ urine sodium [C]
   ■ urine chloride [C]
   ■ urine creatinine [D]
   ■ urine osmolality [C]

Urine biochemistry
Pre-renal failure is more likely with: [C]
• urine sodium < 10 mmol/L
• urine chloride < 10 mmol/L
• urine osmolality > 500 mOsm/kg.

These indices are only valid if patients are not on diuretics and had previously normal renal function.

■ exclude obstruction if it is not clinically obvious: [A]
   ± CT or ultrasound scan [A] – look for hydronephrosis [A]

■ consider inserting a central line [D]

■ consider arranging for a renal biopsy if any of the following are present: [C]
   ■ clinical signs suggestive of primary renal disease, vascular lesions or systemic disease
   ■ no obvious cause of acute renal failure
   ■ suspected acute interstitial nephritis or drug-induced vasculitis
   ■ oligo-anuria thought due to ATN persisting beyond 3 weeks without perpetuating factors.

Note
• 1 in 25 has a clinically important bleed post-biopsy.
• 1 in 150 requires nephrectomy for bleeding lasting > 30 days.

THERAPY

• Treat any potential underlying causes: [D]
   • resuscitate the patient [A]
   • relieve any outflow obstruction [A]
   • stop any nephrotoxic medication. [A]

- Ask for a nephrology opinion. [D]

- The following can help improve urine output. Seek advice if you think they might be necessary. [D]

> **Note**
> None has been shown clearly to reduce the need for dialysis or the risk of dying.

- diuretics [A]

> **High-dose frusemide**
> - Give a loading dose of 120 to 240 mg i.v. slowly.
> - Followed by an infusion of 250 mg in 50 mg 0.9% saline at 10 to 20 mg/h (2 to 4 ml/h), and titre to urine output.
> - If an infusion is impossible, give 120 mg over 1 hour every 6 hours.
> - Reduce the dose if creatinine is falling.
> - Watch for:
>   - seizures
>   - ototoxicity.

- mannitol 20%, single dose of 100 ml for uncorrected hypovolaemia. [C]
- inotropic agents: noradrenaline, dopamine. Patients requiring inotropic support are best monitored in a critical care environment. [D]

> **Noradrenaline**
> - Give via a central line, with ECG monitoring.
> - Make up 4 mg noradrenaline in 50 ml 5.0% glucose.
> - Infuse at a rate of 0.1 to 0.6 µg/kg/min (0.075 ml/kg/h to 0.45 ml/kg/h).
> - Aim to maintain systolic BP >90 mmHg.
> - Watch for:
>   - arrthythmias or cardiac ischaemia
>   - pulmonary oedema
>   - peripheral vasoconstriction. Give an infusion of glyceryl trinitrate 50 mg in 50 ml 0.9% saline at 1 to 10 ml/h if required.

> **Dopamine**
> - Give via a central line, with ECG monitoring.
> - Make up 200 mg dopamine in 50 ml 0.9% saline.
> - Infuse at a rate of 0.5 to 5.0 µg/kg/min (0.0075 ml/kg/h to 0.075 ml/kg/h)
> - Aim to maintain systolic BP >90 mmHg.
> - Watch for:
>   - arrhythmias or cardiac ischaemia
>   - pulmonary oedema.

- Dialyse patients who fail to respond [A] as advised by a specialist. [D]

Common indications include: D
- hyperkalaemia refractory to treatment
- severe or worsening metabolic acidosis
- volume overload
- uraemic pericarditis or encephalopathy.

REVIEW

- Monitor fluid status carefully using daily weights, fluid charts, and invasive monitoring if required.
- Perform regular U&E, creatinine – watch for hyperkalaemia! D
- Restrict water and sodium as necessary.
- Review medication:
  - avoid potential nephrotoxins, e.g. NSAIDs, aminoglycosides D
  - adjust doses of other medications to account for renal insufficiency. D

Fluid balance
Try: D
- input = output + 30 ml/h

Outcomes
- A third require dialysis C – but only 3% require it long-term. C
- Roughly half of patients die, A particularly with a recent MI, stroke or oliguria. B

Expires July 2003   Guideline: Catherine Clase, Chris Ball
CATs: Catherine Clase, Chris Ball, Clare Wotton

36
SICKLE CELL CRISIS

SYMPTOMS AND SIGNS

Common presentations of sickle crises
- Vaso-occlusive: [C]
  - painful
  - priapism. [D]
- Syndromes: [C]
  - acute chest syndrome
  - neurological: stroke, TIA
  - splenic or hepatic sequestration.
- Infection. [C]

Note
Many patients are regular attenders [B] – contact their regular physician and ask how they are normally treated. [D]

Ask about:
- pain and where it is [B]
- potential triggers such as cold weather, exertion, alcohol, pregnancy [C]
- chest pain, fever, dyspnoea, cough [C] (if acute chest syndrome suspected).

Remember to ask about:
- fever and rigors [C] and any possible infection [D]
- abdominal pain. [C]

Look for:
- chest signs [C]
- signs of infection [D]
- focal neurological signs [D]
- an acute abdomen. [C] Ask for a surgical opinion if there are signs of an acute abdomen – it may not be due to the crisis!

Note
- Gallstones are common. [C]
- Investigations including liver function tests and abdominal ultrasound are not very helpful at distinguishing a vaso-occlusive crisis from an acute abdomen. [C]

INVESTIGATIONS

Be guided by the presenting syndrome.

- Blood count, [D] reticulocyte count. [D]
- U&E, creatinine. [D]
- CRP. [D]
- Blood cultures. [D]
- Pulse oximetry – but beware. [C]

> **Note**
> Pulse oximetry is unhelpful in excluding hypoxia in patients with sickle cell disease. [C]

In acute chest syndrome:
- arterial blood gas [D]
- chest X-ray. [D]

Other imaging may be required for acute abdomen and neurological problems. [D]

THERAPY

- Give symptomatic relief and specific therapies where indicated.
- Give oxygen if hypoxic. [A]

In all cases:
- consider broad-spectrum antibiotics [D]
- ensure an adequate fluid intake [D]
- seek expert advice. [D]

Painful crises
Give analgesia: [A]
- Give morphine or diamorphine i.v. or i.m. regularly [A] or via patient-controlled analgesia. [D]
- Avoid regular administration of pethidine. [C]
- Give regular NSAIDs. [A]
- Try TENS if the pain is poorly controlled. [D]

Acute chest syndrome
- Give analgesia. [A]
- Use incentive spirometry. [A]

> **Incentive spirometry**
> Ask patients to breathe as deeply as possible 10 times every 2 hours from 8 a.m. to 10 p.m. and at night if awake until their chest pain settles. [A]

Priapism

- Give analgesia. [A]
- Aspirate the corpus cavernosum and irrigate with dilute adrenaline. [C]
- Proceed to early surgery if there is no resolution. [D]

Priapism
- Following a local anaesthetic injection, aspirate the corpus cavernosum using a 23 G needle, syringe and 3-way tap. [C]
- Then irrigate using 10 ml of 1:1 000 000 solution of adrenaline (i.e. 1 ml of 1:1000 adrenaline in 1 litre 0.9% saline).
- Apply firm pressure for 5 minutes.

Surgery
- Avoid surgery if possible, especially in patients with severe disease. [A]
- If surgery is required, keep it simple. [A]
- Consider transfusing patients before surgery (up to Hb > 10.0 g/dl, is sufficient). [D]

Consider exchange blood transfusions if any of the following are present:
- lung involvement [C]
- sequestration syndromes [D]
- neurological involvement (stroke, TIA, fits). [D]

REVIEW

- Educate your patient about sickle cell crises. [B]
- Give hydroxyurea in severe cases. [A]

Hydroxyurea
- Initial dose 15 mg/kg/day, increase by 5 mg/kg/day every 12 weeks to maximum 35 mg/kg/day, unless marrow depression noted (neutropenia $< 2.0 \times 10^9$/L, reticulocytes or platelets $< 80 \times 10^9$/L, Hb < 4.5 g/dl).
- If this occurs, stop therapy until recovery. Resume at 2.5 mg/kg/day lower.

Consider:
- Depo-Provera contraception for women [A]
- folate [D]
- regular penicillin prophylaxis. [D]

Priapism

Give stilboestrol 5 mg daily by mouth to patients with frequent attacks. [A]

Outcomes

- 30% of patients are admitted to hospital each year [C] – a third of crises happen in only 5%. [B]
- Patients with sickle cell disease die on average in their 40s. [B]
- A third die during acute crises. [B]
- Half of patients with acute chest syndrome have another attack within 10 years. [C]
- Two-thirds of patients with a stroke have another within 10 years. A third die in hospital. [C]
- 40% of men have an episode of priapism a year, but most do not require hospital treatment. [C]

Expires July 2003   Guideline: Chris Ball, Bob Phillips
CATs: Chris Ball, Clare Wotton, Nick Shenker

37
STATUS EPILEPTICUS

SYMPTOMS AND SIGNS

Status epilepticus
Any of:
* continuous seizures for 30 minutes or more.
* two or more seizures without full recovery of consciousness between seizures.

Look for a cause. [D]

Causes of status epilepticus [B]
* discontinued or irregular anticonvulsant use
* alcohol withdrawal
* stroke
* metabolic abnormality or anoxia
* infection
* tumour
* trauma
* drug overdose.

Ask about: [D]
* previous fits
* trauma
* medication
* alcohol and street drugs.

Look for: [D]
* focal neurological signs
* signs of infection
* evidence of drug misuse or overdose.

Exclude:
* hypoxia
* hypoglycaemia.

Note
Think about status in patients in a coma. Signs can be subtle. Look for twitching of extremities, mouth and eyes.

Watch out for pseudoseizures.

> **Pseudoseizures** are more likely if: [C]
> - there is no clear cause for fitting
> - the patient has a psychiatric history
> - the patient is conscious yet having seizures with bilateral motor activity
> - attacks seem atypical
> - the patient resists examination
> - the patient calls out.
>
> Pseudoseizures are less likely if:
> - there are extensor plantars during seizures.

- If in doubt, treat your patient for status epilepticus, but seek expert help, [D] and watch for adverse effects from medication. [C]

INVESTIGATIONS

- Vital signs. [D]
- Pulse oximetry. [D]
- ECG monitoring. [D]

- Rapid blood glucose assay. [A]

- Blood count. [D]
- Urea, electrolytes, creatinine. [D]
- Glucose. [D]
- Liver function tests. [D]
- Calcium, magnesium, phosphate. [D]

- Toxicology screen. [D]
- Anticonvulsant drug levels. [D]

- Arterial blood gases. [D]

Consider requesting an early EEG in unclear cases. [D]

Once your patient is stable, consider:
- head CT or MRI [D]
- lumbar puncture [D]
- EEG. [D]

THERAPY

- Get help. [D]
- Check airway, breathing, circulation. [A]

- Give oxygen. [B]
- Give lorazepam 0.1 mg/kg i.v. at 2 mg/min, [A] or diazepam 0.15 mg/kg i.v. at 5 mg/min. [A] An alternative route is rectally, using larger doses.

If fits continue, try:
- phenobarbital [A] 15 mg/kg i.v. at 100 mg/min
- phenytoin [C] 18 mg/kg i.v. at 50 mg/min.

Phenytoin
- Add 1000 mg phenytoin to at least 100 ml 0.9% saline (max concentration 10 mg/ml).
- Infuse the solution using a syringe driver at no more than 50 mg/min through an in-line filter. [D]
- Flush the line with saline before and after use. [D]
- Arrange for ECG and blood pressure monitoring during infusion.

If fits continue (especially for > 1 hour), intubate and anaesthetize with propofol, [C] midazolam, [D] or thiopental. [D]

REVIEW

Give phenytoin subsequently 100 mg i.v. every 6 to 8 hours, [D] or orally if your patient is fully conscious. Monitor levels.

Outcomes
- Few patients die if treated properly. [B]
- The risk of dying is increased with seizures lasting > 1 hour, anoxia and old age. [B]

Expires July 2003 Guideline: Chris Ball
CATs: Chris Ball, Clare Wotton.

38
STROKE

SYMPTOMS AND SIGNS

Ask about risk factors for stroke:
- hypertension (particularly diastolic > 100 mmHg) [A]
- atrial fibrillation [A]
- diabetes mellitus [A]
- smoking [A]
- high cholesterol [A]
- a previous stroke or TIA [B]
- ischaemic heart disease [A]
- infection within the previous week [B]
- oral contraceptive pill use [B]
- a history of depression. [A]

> **Note**
> 80% of patients have ischaemic strokes, [A] and most involve the anterior circulation. [A]

Look for:
- a carotid bruit, [A] particularly with a history of a TIA or diabetes [A]
- an irregular pulse [B]
- mitral valve prolapse [B] or other heart murmurs. [D]

> **Note**
> The absence of a carotid bruit does not rule out significant carotid artery stenosis. [A]

Assess your patient's functional status, specifically looking for:
- a reduced level of consciousness [A]
- visual neglect [C]
- dysphagia [A]
- a reduction in upper limb motor function [B]
- altered proprioception [B]
- problems standing or walking [B]
- urinary incontinence. [B]

> **Think about other causes of neurological deficits**
> - subarachnoid, extradural, or subdural haemorrhage
> - a space-occupying lesion
> - meningitis or encephalitis
> - hypertensive encephalopathy

- metabolic causes – hypoglycaemia, hyponatraemia
- hypoxia
- trauma.

Classify your patient's type of stroke (based on maximal deficit) using Table 38.1. [A]

Table 38.1   Type of stroke

Stroke subtype	Features
Lacunar infarct (LACI)	Pure motor or sensory stroke, sensorimotor stroke or ataxic hemiparesis
Total anterior circulation infarct (TACI)	A combination of new higher cerebral dysfunction (e.g. dysphasia), homonymous visual field defect, and ipsilateral motor or sensory deficit of at least 2 areas of face, arm and leg
Partial anterior circulation infarct (PACI)	Only 2 of 3 components of TACI; higher cerebral dysfunction alone or with motor/sensory deficit more restricted than for LACI
Posterior circulation infarct (POCI)	Brainstem or cerebellar dysfunction

INVESTIGATIONS

- Blood count. [D]
- U&E, creatinine. [D]
- Glucose. [A]
- Serum lipids. [A]
- ECG. [C]
- Chest X-ray. [D]
- CT or MRI of the head. [B]
- Consider an echocardiogram in young patients. [C]

For patients willing to have carotid endarterectomy, consider:
- carotid ultrasound [A] or MR angiography, [A] followed by angiography if indicated.

THERAPY

Admit your patient to a stroke unit [A] if available and provide intensive physiotherapy [A] and occupational therapy. [A]

Thrombolysis
The benefits of thrombolysis are mixed [A] – it cannot currently be recommended as routine therapy. [D]

Thrombolysis is applicable for patients who understand the risks of intracranial haemorrhage and death, and:
- present within 3 to 6 hours of symptom-onset [C] with a clear neurological deficit [D]
- have a CT scan which excludes a haemorrhagic stroke [A]
- have a neurological deficit that is neither very mild nor very severe [D]
- have no recent trauma, surgery [D] and no active peptic ulcer disease. [D]

REVIEW

- Give patients with a suspected ischaemic stroke aspirin 75 mg daily within 48 hours [A] or as soon as an intracranial haemorrhage has been excluded. [D]
- Consider adding dipyridamole MR 400 mg daily to aspirin. [A]
- Clopidogrel 75 mg daily is an alternative to aspirin. [A]

- Anticoagulate patients with atrial fibrillation. [A]

- Treat risk factors for stroke:
  - Treat hypertension [A] with a diuretic, [A] beta-blocker, [A] ACE inhibitor [A] or calcium-channel blocker. [A]
  - Treat high cholesterol using a statin, [A] e.g. pravastatin 40 mg daily.
  - Optimize diabetes control. [A]
  - Encourage patients to stop smoking [A] and ask nurses [A] and other staff [A] to provide further advice.
    Offer:
    - nicotine patches [A] or gum [A]
    - buproprion. [A]
- Start an ACE inhibitor [A] for patients with:
  - one other cardiovascular risk factor (hypertension, hypercholesterolaemia, low HDL levels, smoking or documented microalbuminuria). [A]

ACE inhibitors
- Monitor the blood pressure for the first dose. [D]
- Increase the dose if patients tolerate it. [A]
- Typical doses:
  - Enalapril 2.5 to 5 mg daily initially, increasing to 10 to 20 mg daily.
  - Perindopril 1 mg daily initially, increasing to 4 to 8 mg daily.
  - Ramipril 1.25 mg daily initially, increasing to 5 mg daily. [A]
- Monitor the renal function. [A]

- Consider performing carotid endarterectomy in patients with carotid stenosis > 50%. [A]

Rehabilitation

> **Note**
> - Half of patients with a first stroke have persistent swallowing problems – watch out for aspiration pneumonia. [A]
> - Watch out for seizures in the first few days. [A]
> - Look for depression – half of patients are clinically depressed at 12 months. [B]

Spasticity
Consider using:
- baclofen [A]
- botulinum toxin for spastic foot [A] or arm [A]
- acupuncture for patients with severe hemiparesis. [A]

Dysphagia
Consider inserting a percutaneous gastrostomy tube (PEG) under antibiotic cover [A] for patients with persistent dysphagia (> 8 days) [A] unless they have: [C]
- GI abnormalities
- ascites or hepatomegaly
- clotting disorders.

Depression
Start fluoxetine 20 mg daily [A] or citalopram 20 mg daily. [A]

Discharge
Consider:
- community rehabilitation [D] with home physiotherapy. [A]

> **Outcomes**
> - A third of patients worsen in the first 4 days. [B]
> - A fifth of patients will have another stroke within 5 years. [B]
> - One in eight patients with a minor stroke will have a major one within 10 years. [A]
> - A third of patients are dead within a year. [B] The risk is lower with a minor stroke or TIA. [A]
>
> | Stroke subtype [A] | Recurrent stroke at 1 year | Death at 1 year |
> | --- | --- | --- |
> | LACI | 9% | 11% |
> | TACI | 6% | 60% |
> | PACI | 17% | 16% |
> | POCI | 20% | 19% |

Expires July 2003 Guideline: Chris Ball
CATs: Chris Ball, Clare Wotton, Nick Shenker

39
SYNCOPE

SYMPTOMS AND SIGNS

Ask about:

- the syncopal episode and what the patient was doing, particularly:
    - any nausea or vomiting before the collapse [A]
    - if it occurred on exertion [B]
    - any tongue biting [C]
    - post-collapse disorientation [C]
    - turning blue [C]

> **Note**
> - A lack of nausea and vomiting increases the risk of an arrhythmia [A]
> - Exertional syncope makes aortic stenosis more likely. [B]
> - Tongue-biting, post-collapse disorientation or turning blue make a seizure more likely. [C]

- any chest pain or dyspnoea [D]
- when the patient last ate [C]
- previous episodes of syncope [A]
- any cardiovascular disease, particularly:
    - known arrhythmias [A]
    - heart failure [A]
    - ischaemic heart disease [A]
    - aortic stenosis [D]
- previous psychiatric problems [C]
- current medication [C]
- a family history of unexplained syncope or sudden death. [C]

> **Causes of syncope include:** [B]
> **Cardiovascular**
> - arrhythmias
> - aortic stenosis
> - myocardial infarction
> - aortic dissection
> - pulmonary embolism.
>
> **Neurological**
> - seizure
> - transient ischaemic attack
> - subclavian steal
> - carotid sinus hypersensitivity
> - vertebro-basilar insufficiency.

Other
- orthostatic hypotension
- drugs
- hypoglycaemia
- situational syncope (micturition, defecation, post-prandial)
- vasovagal attack
- psychogenic.

Look for:
- cardiovascular causes:
    - an irregular [B] or slow-rising pulse [B]
    - apical–carotid delay [B]
    - heart murmurs, particularly aortic stenosis [B]

Note
An irregular pulse makes arrhythmia a more likely cause. [B]

Aortic stenosis [B]
Look for:
+ a slow-rising pulse
± apical–carotid delay.

Listen for: [B]
+ a reduced or absent 2nd heart sound
± a 4th heart sound
± a murmur loudest in late systole
− a murmur radiating to the right carotid.

- injuries [D]

- neurological causes: [B]
    - a decreased level of consciousness
    - any focal neurological signs

- other causes:
    - carotid hypersensitivity – perform carotid sinus massage [D]
    - orthostatic hypotension. [B]

INVESTIGATIONS

- Blood count. [D]
- U&E, creatinine. [D]
- Glucose. [D]
- Cardiac enzymes, [D] including creatine kinase.

> **Note**
> A raised CK makes a tonic–clonic seizure more likely. [A]

■ 12-lead ECG. [B]

> **ECG**
> Look for:
> • ischaemic changes [A]
> • evidence of arrhythmias. [A]

If seizures are suspected, consider:
■ EEG [C]
■ hyperventilation testing. [C]

> **Hyperventilation testing**
> Ask your patient to hyperventilate – if this reproduces two or more symptoms from an attack, seizures are less likely. [C]

If there is no clear cause, consider:
■ an event recorder, [A] or a Holter monitor [B] worn for at least 24 hours and preferably longer. [C]

> **Note**
> The diagnostic or prognostic significance of tilt-table testing [B] or electrophysiological studies [B] is unclear.

THERAPY

• Treat individual diagnoses appropriately. [D]

• Insert a pacemaker in patients with severe recurrent vasovagal syncope. [A] Alternatives include:
  • atenolol [B]
  • paroxetine. [A]

REVIEW

To assess the risk of cardiac arrhythmia or death, [A] use the following guide. Score one point for:
• age > 45
• history of congestive heart failure
• history of ventricular arrhythmias

- abnormal ECG: any of:
  - AF or flutter, or multifocal atrial tachycardia
  - junctional or paced rhythm
  - frequent or repetitive ventricular ectopics (including VT)
  - PR interval < 0.10 mm
  - Mobitz I with other abnormalities, Mobitz II or complete heart block
  - conduction disorder: LAD, BBB, intraventricular delay
  - ventricular hypertrophy
  - old MI.

Then refer to Table 39.1.

Table 39.1   Risk of cardiac arrhythmia or death

Risk factor score	Arrhythmia within a year	Death within a year
3+	45%	27%
2	18%	16%
1	6%	8%
0	3%	1%

Outcomes
- A third of patients have another episode – many within a year. [A]
- A fifth of patients with unexplained syncope have a cardiac arrhythmia. [A] One in 10 is dead within a year [A] – often suddenly. [A]
- If no cardiovascular or neurological cause can be found, recurrences are rare. [A]

Expires July 2003   Guideline: Chris Ball
CATs: Chris Ball, Bob Phillips, Clare Wotton

40
TACHYCARDIAS

SYMPTOMS AND SIGNS

Think about cardiac arrhythmias in patients with:
- palpitations [D]
- dyspnoea [B]
- chest pain [D]
- dizziness or syncope [D]
- cardiac arrest. [D]

Ask about:
- any nausea or vomiting before collapse [A]
- any cardiovascular disease, particularly any:
    - known arrhythmias [A]
    - ischaemic heart disease [D]
- current medication and alcohol use. [D]

> **Note**
> No nausea or vomiting before collapse increases the risk of an arrhythmia. [A]

Look for:
+ an irregular pulse [B]
- cannon waves in the jugular venous pulse (if VT suspected [C])
+ variable amplitude of the first heart sound (if VT suspected [C])
- evidence of cardiovascular decompensation: [B]
    - hypotension
    - pulmonary oedema
    - reduced level of consciousness.

INVESTIGATIONS

- U&E, creatinine. [D]
- Calcium, magnesium. [D]
- Cardiac enzymes. [D]
- Thyroid function tests. [D]
- 12-lead ECG. [A]

Consider further testing if the diagnosis is uncertain and your patient is stable:
- an event recorder [A] or a Holter monitor [B] worn for at least 24 hours and preferably longer [C]
- stress testing to induce the arrhythmia [D]
- an echocardiogram. [D]

Broad-complex tachycardias
- Treat as a ventricular tachycardia until proven otherwise. ᴰ
- Features that favour VT include: ᴰ
  - a history of ischaemic heart disease
  - AV dissociation
  - fusion or capture beats
  - LAD
  - 'RSR¹' pattern in V₁
  - positive concordance across leads.

THERAPY

- Correct any electrolyte abnormality. ᴬ

If uncertain about the source of the arrhythmia:
- Perform carotid sinus massage or ask your patient to perform a Valsalva manoeuvre. ᴰ
- Give adenosine. ᴬ

Adenosine
- Avoid in patients:
  - with asthma
  - on theophyllines, or dipyridamole.
- Use ECG monitoring and have resuscitation equipment available.
- Warn patients about facial flushing, chest discomfort and dyspnoea. ᴬ
- Record the ECG during administration.
- Give 3 mg i.v. rapidly. If unsuccessful after 1 to 2 minutes, try 6 mg, 9 mg then 12 mg. ᴬ
- If the patient has a central line, use it. ᴬ
- Adenosine should:
  - reveal atrial tachycardias
  - terminate junctional re-entrant tachycardia
  - have no effect on ventricular tachycardias.

Acute onset atrial flutter
Control the ventricular rate ᴬ using:
- Digoxin. ᴰ

Digoxin
- Load patients with 500 to 1000 μg in divided doses.
- Give 62.5 to 250 μg daily, based on age, renal function and other medication.
- Measure digoxin levels after 5 days. ᴰ Take the blood test 6 to 10 hours after the last dose.
- Therapeutic range 0.8 to 2.0 ng/ml.

Alternative include:

- Calcium-channel blockers:
  - verapamil 5 mg i.v. over 5 minutes; repeat after 5 minutes to a maximum dose of 20 mg
  - diltiazem 0.25 mg/kg over 2 minutes; repeat at 0.35 mg/kg if no response. [A]

- Beta-blockers:
  - esmolol: [A]
    - load patients with 100 µg/kg/min i.v. over 1 minute
    - followed by 50 µg/kg/min over 4 minutes
    - repeat if there is no effect, and increase the 4-minute infusion by 50 µg/kg/min
  - sotalol: [A]
    - 100 mg i.v. over 5 minutes; or 80 mg orally twice daily.

Consider cardioversion to sinus rhythm [A] if your patient fails to revert spontaneously. [D]

Options include:

- DC cardioversion, [A] particularly if your patient is haemodynamically unstable

---

DC cardioversion

- Patients with acute onset AF or flutter can be cardioverted immediately, [D] but should be started on heparin followed by a month of warfarin. [D]
- In cases of uncertain duration, anticoagulate your patient for a month before and after cardioversion. [C]
- Consider giving an infusion of ibutilide (0.01 mg/kg over 10 minutes) before cardioversion. [A]
- Check your patient has: [D]
  - INR > 2.0 if anticoagulated
  - K > 4.0 mmol/l.
- Arrange for a general anaesthetic for your patient, and ensure your patient is starved for at least 6 hours. [A]
- Cardiovert starting at 100 J; followed by 100 J, 200 J, 300 J, 360 J. [D]

- flecainide [A]

Flecainide

Contraindicated with ischaemic heart disease. [A]

- Intravenous – give 2 mg/kg (to a maximum of 150 mg) over 30 minutes.
- Oral – give 200 mg twice daily, reducing after 3 to 5 days to 50 mg daily.

- ibutilide [A] 0.01 mg/kg to a maximum of 1 mg over 10 minutes
- amiodarone. [A]

Amiodarone
Loading dose:
- Intravenous
  - Preferably via a central line.
  - Give 300 mg (5 mg/kg) in 250 ml 5.0% glucose over 1 hour, followed by 900 mg over 24 hours.

- Oral:
  - Give 200 mg every 8 hours for 1 week, then 200 mg every 12 hours for 1 week, then start maintenance therapy.

Maintenance dose:
- Patients should be given a total loading dose of 4200 mg before starting on maintenance therapy. [D]
- Give 100 to 200 mg daily.

Supraventricular tachycardia
- Try carotid sinus massage or ask your patient to perform a Valsalva manoeuvre. [D]
- Give adenosine. [A]

Adenosine
- Avoid in patients:
  - with asthma
  - on theophyllines, or dipyridamole.
- Use ECG monitoring and have resuscitation equipment available.
- Warn patients about facial flushing, chest discomfort and dyspnoea. [A]
- Record the ECG during administration.
- Give 3 mg rapidly. If unsuccessful after 1 to 2 minutes, try 6 mg, 9 mg then 12 mg. [A]
- If the patient has a central line, use it. [A]
- Adenosine should:
  - reveal atrial tachycardias
  - terminate junctional re-entrant tachycardia
  - have no effect on ventricular tachycardias.

If this fails, consider one of:
- DC cardioversion. [A]

- Calcium channel blockers:
  - diltiazem: 0.25 mg/kg over 2 minutes, repeat at 0.35 mg/kg if no response. [A]

- Beta-blockers:
  - esmolol: [C]
    - load patients with 100 μg/kg/min i.v. over 1 minute
    - followed by 50 μg kg/min over 4 minutes

- repeat if there is no effect, and increase the 4-minute infusion by 50 µg/kg/min
- nadolol: [A] 40 mg orally
- sotalol: [B] 100 mg i.v. over 5 minutes; or 80 mg orally twice daily.

- Propafenone: [B] 150 mg orally three times a day (reduce dose if < 70 kg).

Wolff–Parkinson–White syndrome

> **Note**
> Avoid using digoxin or verapamil – they may exacerbate the arrhythmia. [D]

Terminate the rhythm using any of:
- Adenosine. [D] (See above for further information.)
- Amiodarone. [D] (See above for further information.)
- Flecainide. [D] (See above for further information.)
- Procainamide. [D] Give a bolus of 10 mg per kg at a rate of 100 mg per minute.
- Esmolol. [D] (See above for further information.)
- Diltiazem 0.25 mg/kg over 2 minutes; repeat at 0.35 mg/kg if no response. [A]

Ventricular tachycardia

> **Note**
> Do not treat patients with recent myocardial infarction who have frequent ventricular ectopics with class Ic anti-arrhythmics, e.g. flecainide or encainide. [A]

- Cardiovert patients who are haemodynamically compromised. [A]
- Give amiodarone. [A] (See above for further information.)

Alternatives include:
- sotalol [A] – 100 mg i.v. over 5 minutes, or 80 mg orally twice daily
- procainamide – give a bolus of 10 mg per kg at a rate of 100 mg per minute.

REVIEW

Paroxysmal atrial flutter
- Consider long-term anti-arrhythmic therapy in symptomatic cases. [D]
- Start medication in hospital. [C]

Consider using one of:
- flecainide – at least 50 mg twice daily [A]
- sotalol – at least 120 mg twice daily [A]
- ablation therapy. [D]

Paroxysmal supraventricular tachycardia

- Consider anti-arrhythmic medication for patients with recurrent symptomatic arrhythmias. [D]
- Start medication in hospital. [C]

Consider using one of:
- flecainide – at least 50 mg twice daily [A]
- sotalol 80 mg to 160 mg twice daily [A]
- propafenone 300 mg twice daily [B]
- ablation therapy. [D]

Ventricular arrhythmias

Consider:
- amiodarone [A]
- ablation therapy [D]
- inserting an implantable defibrillator [A] with endocardial leads: [B]
  - Consider adding one of:
    - amiodarone [B]
    - metoprolol [A] 12.5 mg to 50 mg three times a day
    - sotalol [A] 80 mg to 160 mg twice daily.

Implantable defibrillators
Half of patients will receive a shock in the next 2 years. [B]

Outcome
- Only a third of patients with paroxysmal atrial flutter are in sinus rhythm at 2 years. [A]
- 70% of patients with paroxysmal SVT who are not on medication have a recurrent episode within 3 months. [B]
- Half of patients with a ventricular arrhythmia have another episode within 12 months, [B] and around 30% are dead within a year – many suddenly. [B]

Expires July 2003   Guideline: Chris Ball
CATs: Chris Ball, Clare Wotton

41
UPPER GASTROINTESTINAL BLEEDING

SYMPTOMS AND SIGNS

Ask about:

- any haematemesis or melaena before admission and its colour [C] and amount [D]
- other illnesses including:
    - previous peptic ulcers [B]
    - *H. pylori* infection [B]
    - alcohol-related disorders [B]
    - liver cirrhosis, oesophageal varices or portal vein thrombosis [B]
    - renal failure [A]
    - disseminated malignancy [A]
    - heart disease and heart failure [A]
- current medication, particularly:
    - anticoagulants [A]
    - non-steroidal anti-inflammatory drugs (NSAIDs). [A]

Common causes include: [B]
- gastric or duodenal ulcers
- gastric erosions
- varices
- a Mallory–Weiss tear
- oesophagitis.

Rarer causes include:
- tumours [B]
- angiodysplasia.

Look for:

- evidence of acute bleeding: [B]
    + supine tachycardia
    + supine hypotension (systolic blood pressure < 95 mmHg)
    + postural pulse increase of > 30 beats/min or severe dizziness on sitting upright, and if normal then on standing

---

Note
Postural hypotension does not usefully diagnose acute blood loss. [B]

- evidence of anaemia: [A]
    + conjunctival pallor [A]
    + facial pallor [B]
    + palmar pallor [B]
    + dyspnoea [C]

- evidence of cirrhosis, specifically: [A]
  - **+** facial telangiectasia [A]
  - **+** spider naevi [A]
  - **+** abdominal wall veins [A]
  - **+** white nails [A]
  - **+** obesity [A]
  - **+** peripheral oedema. [A]

Risk of cirrhosis [B]

High (> 80%) if:
- all 6 signs present and peripheral oedema
- ≥ 4 signs if no peripheral oedema
- ≥ 3 signs if facial telangiectasia and no peripheral oedema.

Moderate if:
- any other combination.

Low (< 20%) if:
- no facial telangiectasia and ≤ 2 other signs.

Perform a rectal examination and a faecal occult blood test. [A]

Look at the appearance of any vomit or nasogastric aspirate:
- **+** Test it using a gastroccult dipstick. [A]

INVESTIGATIONS

- Blood count. [D]
- Clotting. [A]
- Group and save serum, or cross-match 2 to 6 units depending on blood loss. [D]
- U&E, creatinine. [A]

Urea:creatinine ratio

A urea:creatinine ratio > 100 helps diagnose an upper GI bleed. [A]

- Liver function tests. [A]
- Glucose. [D]
- Blood cultures. [D]
- Arterial blood gases. [D]

Consider inserting:
- a central venous catheter to monitor fluid resuscitation [D]
- a urinary catheter to monitor urine output. [D]

Peptic ulcer disease

Test for *H. pylori* [A] using any of:

- ± CLO test [C]
- ± histology, looking for antral inflammation [C]
- ± urease breath test. [C]

THERAPY

- Resuscitate your patient. [A]
- Insert two large bore i.v. cannulas. [D]
- Give blood if required.
- If PT is prolonged:
  - Give factor concentrate [C] or FFP. [D]
  - Stop any anticoagulants. [C]
  - Consider giving 5 mg vitamin K by slow i.v. infusion. [A]
- Order an endoscopy: [A]
  - urgently [A] to control bleeding
  - to make a diagnosis and determine future risk of bleeding or death. [A]

Endoscopy

Look for evidence of endoscopic stigmata of recent haemorrhage: [A]

- ± blood in the upper GI tract
- ± an adherent clot
- ± a visible or spurting vessel.

Complications of endoscopy such as perforation, aspiration and haemorrhage are very rare. [B]

- While waiting for endoscopy consider giving:
  - somatostatin [A] 6 mg in 500 ml saline i.v. over 24 hours for 5 days
  - octreotide [A]

Octreotide

- Give a bolus of octreotide 50 μg i.v. followed by
- Octreotide 500 μg in 50 ml 0.9% saline at 5 ml/h.

  - terlipressin 2 mg i.v. every 4 hours for up to 72 hours. [A]
- Give thiamine 100 mg [D] i.v. [C] to alcoholics or malnourished patients. [D]
- Discuss any patients likely to rebleed with surgeons and anaesthetists to determine criteria for surgery. [D]

Note

Use the Rockall score [A] (see Table 41.1) to help identify patients at risk of rebleeding or dying.

Table 41.1 Rockall score – rank your patient for risk of rebleeding or dying [A]

	Score 0	Score 1	Score 2	Score 3
Age	• aged < 60	• aged 60 to 79	• aged > 80	

Shock	• pulse < 100
	• systolic b.p.
	  > 100
	  mmHg
		• pulse > 100
		  and systolic
		  BP > 100
		  mmHg
			• pulse > 100
			  and systolic
			  BP < 100
			  mmHg	

Co-morbidity	• no major
	  co-morbidity
			• cardiac
			  failure
			• ischaemic
			  heart disease
			• any other
			  co-morbidity
				• renal failure
				• liver failure
				• disseminated
				  malignancy

Endoscopic stigmata	• none
	• dark spot
	  seen
			• blood in
			  upper GI
			  tract
			• adherent clot
			• visible or
			  spurting
			  vessel	

Diagnosis	• Mallory–Weiss
	  tear
	• no lesion
	  seen and no
	  stigmata of
	  recent
	  haemorrhage
		• all other
		  diagnoses
			• malignancy
			  of upper GI
			  tract	

Pre-endoscopy score	Risk of dying	Post-endoscopy score	Risk of dying	Risk of rebleeding
7	75%	8+	40%	37%
6	62%	7	23%	37%
5	35%	6	12%	27%
4	21%	5	11%	25%
3	12%	4	8%	15%
2	6%	3	2%	12%
1	3%	0 to 2	0%	6%
0	0%			

Peptic ulcers

Arrange for endoscopic haemostasis.

Give:
- a proton pump inhibitor, [A] e.g. omeprazole 40 mg daily
- antacids. [A]

Varices

- Arrange for endoscopic ligation [B] or sclerotherapy [A] within 6 hours. [B]
- Give octreotide or somatostatin. [A]

> **Somatostatin**
> Somatostatin 6 mg in 500 ml saline i.v. over 24 hours for 5 days.

> **Octreotide**
> Octreotide 500 µg in 50 ml 0.9% saline at 50 µg per hour (i.e. 5 ml/h.)

Consider:
- balloon tamponade [A] for patients who do not stop bleeding [D]
- transjugular intrahepatic portosystemic shunts (TIPS). [D]

REVIEW

Monitor: [D]
- vital signs and urine output
- blood count
- clotting
- electrolytes.

Consider:
- iron supplements, [B] e.g. ferrous sulphate 200 mg three time a day [D]
- tranexamic acid [A] for patients likely to rebleed (3 to 6 g i.v. for 3 days, followed by 3 to 6 g orally for 3 to 5 days). [D]

Patients with a Mallory–Weiss tear or an ulcer can start eating immediately on recovery from endoscopy. [D]

Rebleeding

Perform repeat endoscopy on patients with: [A]
- vomiting of fresh blood
- hypotension and melaena
- requirement for 4 units of blood in the first 72 hours after endoscopic treatment.

Consider surgery if there is persistent or recurrent haemorrhage despite endoscopic therapy. [D]

Ulcers and erosions
- A routine repeat endoscopy is not necessary. [D]
- Advise patients to stop smoking. [B]
- Stop NSAIDs. [A] If patients need to continue, consider:
  - COX-2 inhibitors, e.g. rofecoxib [A] 12.5 to 25 mg daily or celecoxib [B]
  - topical NSAIDs [B]
  - ibuprofen [B] at the lowest possible dose [B]
  - adding in regular omeprazole 40 mg daily [A] or misoprostol [A] 200 µg 2 to 4 times daily. [D]
- Give *H. pylori* eradication therapy [A] using triple therapy: [B]
  - a proton-pump inhibitor plus any two of amoxicillin, clarithromycin or a nitroimidazole [B]
  - a bismuth compound plus a nitroimidazole plus tetracycline. [B]

Sample triple therapy regimen: a 7-day course
- omeprazole 20 mg twice daily
- clarithromycin 500 mg twice daily
- amoxicillin 1 g twice daily.

- Continue proton-pump inhibitors long-term. [A]

Varices
- Arrange for endoscopic ligation [A] or sclerotherapy [A] until varices are obliterated.
- Give beta-blockers, [A] e.g. propranolol MR 80 mg daily or isosorbide mononitrate MR [A] 60 mg daily.

Outcomes
- One in seven patients dies in hospital [A] – one in 15 from further bleeding.
- Peptic ulcers heal slowly and a third of patients have a relapse within a year. [B]
- A third of patients with varices rebleed within 1 year. [B] A third are dead within 2 months. [A]

Expires July 2003   Guideline: Alan Townsend, Chris Ball
CATs: Alan Townsend, Chris Ball, Clare Wotton

APPENDIX 1
LEVELS OF EVIDENCE

What are we to do when the irresistible force of the need to offer clinical advice meets with the immovable object of flawed evidence? All we can do is our best: give the advice, but alert the advisees to the flaws in the evidence on which it is based.

The ancestor of these levels was created by Suzanne Fletcher and Dave Sackett 20 years ago when they were working for the Canadian Task Force on the Periodic Health Examination.[i] They generated 'levels of evidence' for ranking the validity of evidence about the value of preventive manoeuvres, and then tied them as 'grades of recommendations' to the advice given in the report.

The levels have evolved over the ensuing years, most notably as the basis for recommendations about the use of antithrombotic agents,[ii] have grown increasingly sophisticated,[iii] and have even started to appear in a new generation of evidence-based textbooks that announce, in bold marginal icons, the grade of each recommendation that appears in the texts in bold icons.[iv]

However, their orientation remained therapeutic/preventive, and when a group of members of the Centre for Evidence-based Medicine embarked on creating *EBOC*, the need for levels and grades for diagnosis, prognosis, and harm became overwhelming and the current version (Table A1.1) appears here. This is the work of Chris Ball, Dave Sackett, Bob Phillips, Brian Haynes, and Sharon Straus, with lots of encouragement and advice from their colleagues.

Periodic updates will appear at http://cebm.jr2.ox.ac.uk/docs/levels.html#levels, and readers are invited to suggest ways in which they might be improved or further developed.

A cautionary note: these levels and grades speak only to the validity of evidence about prevention, diagnosis, prognosis, therapy, and harm. Other strategies, described elsewhere in the Centre's pages, must be applied to the evidence in order to generate clinically useful measures of its potential clinical implications and to incorporate vital patient values into the ultimate decisions.

---

[i] Canadian Task Force on the Periodic Health Examination: The periodic health examination. CMAJ 1979; 121: 1193–1254.

[ii] Sacket DL. Rules of evidence and clinical recommendations on use of antithrombotic agents. Chest 1986; 89 (2 suppl.): 2S–3S.

[iii] Cook DJ, Guyatt GH, Laupacis A, Sackett DL, Goldberg RJ. Clinical recommendations using levels of evidence for antithrombotic agents. Chest 1995; 108 (4 suppl): 227S–230S.

[iv] Yusuf S, Cairns JA, Camm AJ, Fallen EL, Gersh BJ. Evidence-Based Cardiology. London: BMJ Publishing Group; 1998.

NOTES

- Recommendations based on this approach apply to 'average' patients and may need to be modified in light of an individual patient's unique biology (risk, responsiveness, etc.) and preferences about the care they receive.
- Users can add a minus-sign '–' to denote the level of evidence that fails to provide a conclusive answer because of:
  - *either* a single result with a wide Confidence Interval (such that, for example, an ARR in an RCT is not statistically significant but the confidence intervals fail to exclude clinically important benefit or harm)
  - *or* a Systematic Review with troublesome (and statistically significant) heterogeneity.
- Such evidence is inconclusive, and therefore can only generate Grade D recommendations.

Table A1.1 Levels of evidence

Grade of recommendation	Level of evidence	Therapy/prevention, aetiology/harm	Prognosis
A	1a	SR (with homogeneity[1]) of RCTs	SR (with homogeneity[1]) of inception cohort studies; or a CPG[2] validated on a test set
	1b	Individual RCT (with narrow Confidence Interval[3])	Individual inception cohort study with ≥ 80% follow-up
	1c	All or none[5]	All or none case-series
B	2a	SR (with homogeneity[1]) of cohort studies	SR (with homogeneity[1]) of either retrospective cohort studies or untreated control groups in RCTs
	2b	Individual cohort study (including low quality RCT; e.g. < 80% follow-up)	Retrospective cohort study or follow-up of untreated control patients in an RCT; or CPG not validated in a test set
	2c	'Outcomes' research	Outcomes research
	3a	SR (with homogeneity[1]) of case-control studies	
B	3b	Individual case-control study	

Diagnosis	Economic analysis
SR (with homogeneity[1]) of Level 1 diagnostic studies; or a CPG[2] validated on a test set	SR (with homogeneity[1]) of Level 1 economic studies
Independent blind comparison of patients from an *appropriate* spectrum[4] of patients, all of whom have undergone both the diagnostic test and the reference standard	Analysis comparing all (critically validated) alternative outcomes against appropriate cost measurement, and including a sensitivity analysis incorporating clinically sensible variations in important variables
Absolute SpPins and SnNouts[6]	Clearly as good or better[7] but cheaper. Clearly as bad or worse but more expensive. Clearly better or worse at the same cost
SR (with homogeneity[1]) of Level ≥ 2 diagnostic studies	SR (with (homogeneity[1]) of Level ≥ 2 economic studies
Any of: • Independent blind or objective comparison • Study performed in a set of non-consecutive patients, or confined to a narrow spectrum of study individuals (or both), all of whom have undergone both the diagnostic test and the reference standard • A diagnostic CPG not validated in a test set	Analysis comparing a limited number of alternative outcomes against appropriate cost measurement, and including a sensitivity analysis incorporating clinically sensible variations in important variables
Independent blind or objective comparison of an appropriate spectrum[4] but the reference standard was not applied to all study patients	Analysis without accurate cost measurement, but including a sensitivity analysis incorporating clinically sensible variations in important variables

Table A1.1 *(Continued)*

Grade of recommendation	Level of evidence	Therapy/prevention, aetiology/harm	Prognosis
	4	Case-series (and poor quality cohort and case-control studies[8])	Case-series (and poor quality prognostic cohort studies[9])
C			
	5	Expert opinion without explicit critical appraisal, or based on physiology, bench research or 'first principles'	Expert opinion without explicit critical appraisal, or based on physiology, bench research or 'first principles'
D			

1. By homogeneity we mean a systematic review that is free of worrisome variations (heterogeneity) in the directions and degrees of results between individual studies. Not all systematic reviews with statistically significant heterogeneity need be worrisome, and not all worrisome heterogeneity need be statistically significant. As noted above, studies, displaying worrisome heterogeneity should be tagged with a '–' at the end of their designated level.
2. Clinical Practice Guide.
3. See Notes above for advice on how to understand, rate and use trials or other studies with wide Confidence Intervals.
4. An appropriate spectrum is a cohort of patients who would normally be tested for the target disorder. An inappropriate spectrum compares patients already known to have the target disorder with patients diagnosed with another condition.
5. Met when *all* patients died before the Rx became available, but some now survive on it; or when some patients died before the Rx became available, but *none* now die on it.
6. An 'Absolute SpPin' is a diagnostic finding whose Specificity is so high that a Positive result rules-*in* the diagnosis. An 'Absolute SnNout' is a diagnostic finding whose Sensitivity is so high that a Negative result rules-*out* the diagnosis.
7. Good, better, bad and worse refer to the comparisons between treatments in terms of their clinical risks and benefits.
8. By poor quality cohort study we mean one that failed to clearly define comparison groups and/or failed to measure exposures and outcomes in the same (preferably blinded) objective way in both exposed and non-exposed individuals and/or failed to

Diagnosis	Economic analysis
Any of: • Reference standard was unobjective, unblinded or not independent • Positive and negative tests were verified using separate reference standards • Study was performed in an inappropriate spectrum[4] of patients	Analysis with no sensitivity analysis
Expert opinion without explicit critical appraisal, or based on physiology, bench research or 'first principles'	Expert opinion without explicit critical apprasial, or based on economic theory

identify or appropriately control known confounders and/or failed to carry out a sufficiently long and complete follow-up of patients. By poor quality case-control study we mean one that failed to clearly define comparison groups and/or failed to measure exposures and outcomes in the same (preferably blinded) objective way in both cases and controls and/or failed to identify or appropriately control known confounders.

9. By poor quality prognostic cohort study we mean one in which sampling was biased in favour of patients who already had the target outcome, or the measurement of outcomes was accomplished in < 80% of study patients, or outcomes were determined in an unblinded, non-objective way, or there was no correction for confounding factors.

APPENDIX 2
ABBREVIATIONS USED

ACE inhibitors	angiotension converting enzyme inhibitors
AF	atrial fibrillation
ANA	anti-nuclear antibodies
ANCA	anti-neutrophilic cytoplasmic antibodies
anti-dsDNA	anti-double-stranded DNA antibodies
anti-GBM	anti-glomerular basement membrane antibodies
ARF	acute renal failure
ARR	absolute risk reduction
AST	aspartate transaminase
ATN	acute tubular necrosis
AV	atrioventricular
BBB	bundle branch block
b.d.	twice daily (*bis die*)
BMI	body mass index
BP	blood pressure
CABG	coronary artery bypass grafting
CEA	carcinoembryonic antigen
CK	creatine kinase
Cl	chloride
CLL	chronic lymphocytic leukaemia
CNS	central nervous system
CO	carbon monoxide
COPD	chronic obstructive pulmonary disease
CPAP	continuous positive airway pressure
CPR	cardiopulmonary resuscitation
Cr	creatinine
CrCl	creatinine clearance
CRP	C-reactive protein
CT	computed tomography
CVP	central venous pressure
DKA	diabetic ketoacidosis
DVT	deep vein thrombosis
ECG	electrocardiogram
EEG	electroencephalogram
ESR	erythrocyte sedimentation rate
FEV_1	forced expiratory volume at 1 second
FFP	fresh frozen plasma
G	gauge
GCS	Glasgow Coma Scale
GI	gastrointestinal
GU	genitourinary
h	hours

HCO_3	bicarbonate
HUS	haemolytic uraemic syndrome
IBD	inflammatory bowel disease
ICU	intensive care unit
i.m.	intramuscular
INR	international normalized ratio
i.v.	intravenous
JVP	jugular venous pressure
K	potassium
LAD	left axis deviation
LDH	lactate dehydrogenase
MCV	mean cell volume
MI	mycardial infarction
min	minutes
MMA	methylmalonic acid
MRI	magnetic resonance imaging
MSU	midstream urine
Na	sodium
NSAIDs	non-steroidal anti-inflammatory drugs
PCR	polymerase chain reaction
PE	pulmonary embolism
PEG	percutaneous endoscopic gastrostomy
PT	prothrombin time
PTCA	percutaneous transluminal coronary angioplasty
q.d.s.	four times daily (*quarter die sumendus*)
RCT	randomized controlled trial
RDW	red cell distribution width
s.c.	subcutaneously
SIADH	syndrome of inappropriate antidiuretic hormone
SLE	systemic lupus erythematosus
SR	systematic review
SVT	supraventricular tachycardia
TB	tuberculosis
t.d.s	three times daily (*ter die sumendus*)
TIA	transient ischaemic attack
TTP	thrombotic thrombocytopenic purpura
UA	unstable angina
U&E	urea and electrolytes
VF	ventricular fibrillation
VT	ventricular tachycardia

LEVELS OF EVIDENCE SUMMARY

Grade of Recommendation	Level of Evidence	Therapy
[A]	1a	Systematic review of RCTs
	1b	Single RCT
	1c	'All-or-none'
[B]	2a	Systematic review of cohort studies
	2b	Cohort study or poor RCT
	2c	'Outcomes' research
	3a	Systematic review of case-control studies
	3b	Case-control study
[C]	4	Case-series
[D]	5	Expert opinion, physiology, bench research